THE
BLOOD
SUGAR
SOLUTION
COOKBOOK

WITHDRAWN

ALSO BY MARK HYMAN, MD

The Blood Sugar Solution

UltraPrevention

UltraMetabolism

The Five Forces of Wellness (CD)

The UltraMetabolism Cookbook

The UltraThyroid Solution

The UltraSimple Diet

The UltraSimple Challenge (DVD)

The UltraMind Solution

Six Weeks to an UltraMind (CD)

UltraCalm (CD)

THE
BLOOD
SUGAR
SOLUTION
COOKBOOK

More than 175 Ultra-Tasty Recipes
for Total Health and Weight Loss

Mark Hyman, MD

LITTLE, BROWN AND COMPANY
New York   Boston   London

This book is intended to supplement, not replace, the advice of a trained health professional.
If you know or suspect that you have a health problem, you should consult a health professional.
The author and publisher specifically disclaim any liability, loss, or risk, personal or otherwise,
that is incurred as a consequence, directly or indirectly, of the use and application of any
of the contents of this book.

Copyright © 2013 by Hyman Enterprises LLC

All rights reserved. In accordance with the U.S. Copyright Act of 1976, the scanning, uploading,
and electronic sharing of any part of this book without the permission of the publisher constitute
unlawful piracy and theft of the author's intellectual property. If you would like to use material
from the book (other than for review purposes), prior written permission must be obtained
by contacting the publisher at permissions@hbgusa.com. Thank you for your support of
the author's rights.

Little, Brown and Company
Hachette Book Group
237 Park Avenue, New York, NY 10017
littlebrown.com

First Edition: February 2013

Little, Brown and Company is a division of Hachette Book Group, Inc. The Little, Brown name
and logo are trademarks of Hachette Book Group, Inc.

The publisher is not responsible for websites (or their content) that are not owned by the publisher.

The Hachette Speakers Bureau provides a wide range of authors for speaking events. To find out
more, go to hachettespeakersbureau.com or call (866) 376-6591.

Photographs by Jonathan Heindemause

ISBN 978-0-316-24819-8
LCCN 2012953741

10 9 8 7 6 5 4 3 2 1

RRD-C

Printed in the United States of America

For all those who seek to take back their health

Contents

PART I

THE BASICS

PART II

THE RECIPES

Tools and Resources for the Blood Sugar Solution

This cookbook is designed to be used alone, and if you follow the recipes and the program, it will work on its own. But there is so much more to share and explain about how and why this program works, and additional tools and resources to help you succeed. I encourage you to review my book *The Blood Sugar Solution,* join our online community, and get free access to hundreds of videos, including my cooking videos. You will also get access to health-tracking tools to track your diet, exercise, measurements, and lab tests, as well as a guide to what tests to take, tips on how to work with your doctor to get what you need, information about supplements, and more. You can access nutrition and life coaching, a rich assortment of articles and educational materials, and even additional recipes. In addition, the online UltraWellness Community is made up of tens of thousands of people just like you who help guide, support, and encourage one another as they work through many of the same issues. And for those who need a bit more support, I lead a 12-week online course on the Blood Sugar Solution—go to bloodsugarsolution.com to learn more. My goal is for you to say, "I didn't know I was feeling so bad until I started feeling so good."

Cooking Is a Revolutionary Act*

The cure for what ails us—both in our bodies and in our nation—can be found in the kitchen. It is a place to rebuild community and connection, strengthen bonds with family and friends, teach life-giving skills to our children, enrich and nourish our bodies and our souls. Yet, in the twenty-first century, our kitchens (and our taste buds) have been hijacked by the food industry. In 1900 only 2 percent of meals were eaten outside of the home; today that number is over 50 percent.

The foodlike substances proffered by the industrial food system trick our taste buds into momentary pleasure. But our biology rejects the junk forced on our genes and on our hormonal and biochemical pathways. Your tongue can be fooled and your brain can become addicted to the slick combinations of fat, sugar, and salt pumped into factory-made foods, but your biochemistry cannot handle these foods, and the result is the disaster we have in America today—70 percent of us are overweight, and obesity rates are expected to top 42 percent by the end of the next decade (up from only 13 percent in 1960).

Today one in two Americans has either pre-diabetes or diabetes. In less than a decade the rate of pre-diabetes or diabetes in teenagers has risen from 9 percent to 23 percent. Really? Almost one in four kids has pre-diabetes or type 2 diabetes? Yes, and perhaps even more shocking,

---

* Pilar Gerasimo and her *101 Revolutionary Ways to Be Healthy* inspired the idea that cooking is a revolutionary act. To learn the other 100 revolutionary ways to be healthy, go to revolutionaryact.com or check out the app.

37 percent of kids at a *normal weight* have one or more cardiovascular risk factors such as high blood pressure, high cholesterol, or high blood sugar, because even though factory food doesn't necessarily make you fat, it does make you sick! The food industry taxes our health and mortgages our children's futures. Obese children will earn less, suffer more, and die younger.

It is time to take back our kitchens and our homes. Transforming the food industry seems like a gigantic undertaking, but it is in fact an easy fix. The solution is in our shopping carts, our refrigerators, and our cupboards—and on our dining room tables. This is where the power is. It is the hundreds of small choices you make every day, choices that will topple the monolithic food industry.

We need a revolution. Cooking real food is a revolutionary act. We have lost the means to care for ourselves. We have now raised the second generation of Americans who don't know how to cook. The average child in America doesn't know how to identify even the most basic vegetables and fruit; our kids don't know where their food comes from or even that it grows on a farm. Cooking means microwaving. Food comes in boxes, plastic bags, and cans. Reading labels is supremely unhelpful in identifying the source of most foods—the ingredients are mostly factory-made science projects with a remote and unrecognizable lineage to real food.

We are brainwashed into thinking that cooking real food costs too much, is too hard, and takes too long. Hence, we rely on inexpensive convenience foods. But these aren't so convenient when we become dependent on hundreds of dollars of medication a month, when we can't work because we are sick and fat and sluggish, or when we feel so bad we can't enjoy life anymore. The average American spends eight hours a day in front of a screen (mostly the television) and spends more time watching cooking shows than actually cooking.

Convenience is killing us.

In fact, real food can be inexpensive. Choosing simple ingredients, cooking from scratch, shopping at discount club stores, and getting produce from community supported agriculture associations (CSAs), community gardens, or co-ops all build health and community and save money. Europeans spend nearly 20 percent of their income on food, Americans only about 9 percent. Food is the best investment in your health.

I believe in the power of collective intelligence. Within my community are hundreds, if not thousands, of unheralded chefs experimenting with food and creating extraordinary meals and recipes. Within our individual and our national communities is the cure for what ails us. We are the answer. We are the revolutionaries who will change the face of food in America and around the world. *The Blood Sugar Solution Cookbook* is the product of this collective intelligence. Truly, the community is the cure!

Yes, we need to change policy in order to change the food we grow and to subsidize real food instead of the walls of processed fat, sugar, flour, and trans fats that line our grocery and convenience stores. Yes, we need to end food marketing to children. We need to make schools safe zones for kids with only those products and activities that support healthy minds and bodies. There is no room for junk food or factory foods in schools. Period. Yes, we need all that and more to take back our kitchens and our health. But each of us can start at home with a kitchen makeover. Three simple actions can change everything:

1. Do a fridge makeover.
2. Do a pantry makeover.
3. Do a shopping cart makeover.

This book gives you advice on what to keep and what to discard from your fridge, pantry, and shopping cart. It also provides recipes—gathered from our own community of health and cooking revolutionaries—to delight your palate, stimulate your senses, and nourish your body and soul. The recipes are designed to be made, shared, and enjoyed with friends and family. Think of this book as a roadmap to pleasure and health.

Once you have taken back your kitchen, then you can start something really revolutionary. Find eight (or so) people you would love to know better or spend more time with. Invite them to start a supper club—once a week or once a month. Rotate dinners at one another's houses. Share the cooking by creating a potluck, or take turns choosing some favorite recipes from this cookbook and preparing a feast for all. At each dinner pick a topic—about food, health, or community—to discuss. Then let the juices flow. The stew of food and friendship will nourish you deeply.

In this way—one by one, kitchen by kitchen, community by community—we will take back our health together!

PART I

THE BASICS

1

What Is the Blood Sugar Solution?

My book *The Blood Sugar Solution* is an owner's manual for personal health and a manifesto for us all to take back our health. First, it provides a step-by-step, goof-proof plan to reverse the root causes of diabetes and obesity—what I call *diabesity*. Next, it provides a roadmap for us to get healthy together—because getting healthy is a team sport. Finally, it is a manifesto motivating us to take back our health in our kitchens, homes, schools, workplaces, faith-based communities, and even in our media, our food system, our health-care system, and our democracy. A tall order to be sure, but one that is necessary if we are to have a sustainable future— for ourselves, our children, our economy, and the environment.

The Blood Sugar Solution is all about the root causes of chronic disease— and one of the major culprits is poor nutrition. The fundamental idea revolutionizing nutrition science is this: *food is not just calories; it is information.* And with the right information you can upgrade your biological software in real time, literally with every bite. Food is medicine. In fact, what you put on your fork is more powerful than anything you will ever find in a pill bottle. The recipes in this book were created based on the guidelines in *The Blood Sugar Solution,* a six-week plan designed to reverse diabesity. I have included recipes designed to be used when the six weeks are over, during what I call the "reintroduction phase." I have also added a few special low-glycemic desserts (low glycemic refers to foods that don't raise your blood sugar as much or as fast as high glycemic foods), which can be enjoyed at the end of the first six weeks of the plan as occasional treats.

DO I HAVE DIABESITY?

Diabesity refers to the continuum of blood sugar and insulin imbalance that causes everything from mild weight problems and a little belly fat to pre-diabetes to full-blown type 2 diabetes. It affects one in two Americans, one in four African Americans, one in four Medicare patients, and one in four teenagers. It is a global problem—80 percent of the world's diabetics live in developing countries. And it affects skinny people, too! In fact 37 percent of skinny kids and 23 percent of skinny adults (only 35 percent of Americans are considered of normal weight) have diabesity—they look skinny but are metabolically fat. Doctors call it "metabolically obese normal weight." I call it the "skinny fat syndrome." Indeed, 90 percent of people with diabesity are *not* diagnosed. In other words, you probably have it and don't know it.

Take this short quiz to see if you might have diabesity, and then the extended quiz on page 10. You can also take the whole quiz at bloodsugarsolution.com/take-the-diabesity-quiz/.

Do I Have Diabesity?

If you answer "yes" to any of these questions, you may already have diabesity or are headed in that direction. If so, continue on to the Comprehensive Diabesity Quiz on page 10.

- Do you have a family history of diabetes, heart disease, or obesity?

  Yes ___ No ___

- Are you of nonwhite ancestry (African, Asian, Native American, Pacific Islander, Hispanic, Indian, Middle Eastern)?   Yes ___ No ___

- Are you overweight (body mass index [BMI] over 25)? See page 8 to calculate your BMI based on weight and height.   Yes ___ No ___

- Do you have extra belly fat? Is your waist circumference greater than 35 inches for women or greater than 40 inches for men?

  Yes ___ No ___

- Do you crave sugar and refined carbohydrates? Yes ___ No ___

- Do you have trouble losing weight on a low-fat diet? Yes ___ No ___

- Has your doctor told you that your blood sugar is a little high (greater than 100 mg/dl) or have you actually been diagnosed with insulin resistance, pre-diabetes, or diabetes? Yes ___ No ___

- Do you have high levels of triglycerides (over 100 mg/dl) or low HDL (good) cholesterol (<50 mg/dl)? Yes ___ No ___

- Do you have heart disease? Yes ___ No ___

- Do you have high blood pressure? Yes ___ No ___

- Are you inactive (less than 30 minutes of exercise 4 times a week)? Yes ___ No ___

- Do you suffer from infertility, low sex drive, or sexual dysfunction? Yes ___ No ___

- For women: Have you had gestational diabetes or polycystic ovarian syndrome? Yes ___ No ___

The Blood Sugar Solution translates scientific research into practical recommendations for anyone who wants to get and stay healthy. Soon you will start on the path toward balancing your insulin. But first you need to take some baseline measurements, a quiz, and a few tests to determine which version of the program you should be following, and which recipes in this book are right for you.

THE BASIC AND ADVANCED PLANS

There are two versions of the program. The one you need depends on your score on the comprehensive diabesity quiz. The **Basic Plan** can be followed by anyone. It balances your blood sugar, reduces insulin spikes, balances hormones, cools off inflammation, helps improve digestion, boosts your metabolism, enhances detoxification, and calms your mind and nervous system. Eighty percent of you following the Basic Plan will have all the tools you need to heal from diabesity and take control of your health.

The **Advanced Plan** is designed for people with more severe cases of diabesity, including those who have been diagnosed with type 2 diabetes. Some of us are genetically more susceptible to becoming insulin resistant and pump out much more insulin in response to a given sugar load, even if we are thin. The genomic revolution and our understanding of the various factors that create imbalances in our metabolism force us to move beyond the one-size-fits-all prescriptions of the past into personalized medicine and health.

If you qualify for the Advanced Plan you will need to take an additional set of supplements (see my book *The Blood Sugar Solution* or visit bloodsugarsolution.com/diabesity-supplements) and to make a few extra dietary changes.

To determine which plan is best for you and effectively track your progress, you need to complete three action steps: gather your measurements, take the quiz on page 10, and get tested.

START A JOURNAL NOW

Before you start the program, I want you to start keeping a journal. Journaling is an excellent way to get in touch with your inner guidance system, to break the cycle of mindless eating and activity, to be honest and accountable and present to yourself. You might overeat because something is eating you, or stuff yourself with food in order to stuff your feelings away. If you use food to block feelings, you can instead use words to block food. You can write in order to better metabolize your feelings so they don't end up driving unconscious choices or overeating. A diet of words and self-exploration often results in weight loss.

You can also use the journal to track your daily food intake, your exercise, sleep, symptoms, and your "numbers," including weight, waist size, and lab tests. Watching how you feel as you alter your food intake, begin taking supplements, and start to exercise more is like "innercise" that will strengthen your capacity for creating high-level wellness and wholeness.

GATHER AND RECORD YOUR BODY MEASUREMENTS

You can quickly gather and track critical information about your health with four simple, easy-to-obtain measurements that will speak volumes about your health and metabolism. Here is what to measure and how to measure it. (You can find special health trackers and online versions of these tools at bloodsugarsolution.com/health-tracker.)

YOUR WEIGHT

- Weigh yourself first thing in the morning without clothes and after going to the bathroom. Track your weight weekly in your journal.

YOUR HEIGHT

- Measure yourself in feet and inches. Write it in your journal.

YOUR WAIST SIZE

- Measure the widest point around your belly button. Track this measurement weekly in your journal.

YOUR BLOOD PRESSURE

- Buy a home blood pressure cuff or go to a drugstore that measures blood pressure for free, or ask your doctor to measure it.
- Measure your blood pressure first thing in the morning, before you start your daily activities. Ideal blood pressure is less than 115/75. Over 140/90 is significantly elevated.
- Track your blood pressure weekly in your journal.

Once you have these critical measurements you can determine other key numbers.

1. YOUR BODY MASS INDEX (BMI)

* Your BMI is your weight in kilograms divided by your height in meters squared. For ease of calculation, use our online calculator at blood-sugarsolution.com/tracking-tools. Or use this calculation: BMI = weight in pounds times 703, divided by height in inches squared. For example, I weigh 185 pounds and am 75 inches tall, so my BMI is $185 \times 703/75^2 = 23$.

* This gives you a way to track whether you are normal weight, overweight, or obese. Normal BMI is less than 25, overweight is 26 to 29, and obese is over 30. However, you should take into account your waist size as well. If you weigh a lot but are a muscular bodybuilder with a small waist, you could be healthy. If you have skinny arms and legs and a skinny butt but a potbelly, you might have a normal BMI but be at risk for diabesity. Furthermore, certain ethnic groups—such as Asians, Hispanics, Pacific Islanders, Inuit, Indians, and Middle Easterners—have diabesity at much lower BMIs.

* Track your BMI weekly in your journal along with your other measurements.

2. YOUR WAIST-TO-HEIGHT RATIO

* To calculate this, divide your waist measurement by your height in inches, and then move the decimal point two places to the right. See the chart opposite to interpret your waist-to-height ratio or go to bloodsugarsolution.com and enter your height and weight online. It will then be automatically calculated for you.

* This measurement tells whether you are fat around the middle. (If you stand sideways while looking in the mirror and have a big belly, or if you can't see your toes when standing up, then you have a problem.)

* This number is a better predictor of diabesity, heart disease, and risk of death than almost any other number. It is also easier to calculate.

* Measure this weekly while on the program and record it in your journal. Once you have gone off the program, you can measure it once a month.

Waist-to-Height Table

WOMEN

- Ratio <35: abnormally slim to underweight
- Ratio 35–41: extremely slim
- Ratio 42–45: slender and healthy
- Ratio 46–48: healthy, normal weight
- Ratio 49–53: overweight
- Ratio 54–58: extremely overweight/obese
- Ratio >58: highly obese

MEN

- Ratio <35: abnormally slim to underweight
- Ratio 35–42: extremely slim
- Ratio 43–45: slender and healthy
- Ratio 46–52: healthy, normal weight
- Ratio 53–57: overweight
- Ratio 58–63: extremely overweight/obese
- Ratio >63: highly obese

Go to bloodsugarsolution.com/health-tracker to learn more about our online tracking tools. They can help you track all of your quiz scores, body measurements, and blood test results, as well as your daily experiences, thoughts, and feelings so you can easily measure your progress over time. Tracking your progress will benefit you, but if you share your progress at bloodsugarsolution.com, you can also be part of our patient-driven research program and help transform health care to improve the health of others.

Take the Comprehensive Diabesity Quiz

Now that you have recorded your BMI and waist-to-height ratio, you are ready to find out whether you should go on the Basic or Advanced Plan. At the beginning of this chapter you took a simple screening quiz to see if you might have diabesity. Now you can take a closer look at the severity of your problem. Take the quiz below. Score one point for each of the questions you answer "yes" to.

Comprehensive Diabesity Quiz	YES	NO
Do you ever get an urge for something sweet, give in to it, experience a brief "sugar high," and later crash into the "sugar blues"?		
Did your doctor ever tell you that your blood sugar was "a little high"?		
Would you describe yourself as an inactive person?		
If you go more than a few hours between meals, do you get irritable, anxious, tired, jittery, or have headaches intermittently throughout the day — and then feel better after you've eaten?		
Do you feel shaky 2–3 hours after a meal?		
Do you have trouble losing weight on a low-fat diet?		
If you miss a meal, do you feel cranky, irritable, weak, or tired?		
If you have a muffin, a bagel, cereal, pancakes, or other carbs for breakfast, is your eating out of control all day?		
Do you feel as though you can't stop eating once you start eating sweets or carbohydrates?		
Does a bowl of pasta or potatoes put you right to sleep, but a meal of fish or meat and vegetables makes you feel good?		
Do you go straight for the bread basket at restaurants?		
Do you get heart palpitations after eating sweets?		
Do you tend to retain water after eating salty foods?		
If you skip breakfast, are you likely to have a panic attack in the afternoon?		
Do you absolutely, positively have to have your cup of coffee in the morning in order to get yourself going?		
Do you often get moody, impatient, or anxious?		
Have you been having any problems lately with your memory and concentration?		

continues on next page

Comprehensive Diabesity Quiz (*continued*)	YES	NO
Do you feel calmer after you eat?		
Do you get tired a few hours after eating?		
Do you get night sweats (even if you are a man)?		
Do you feel the need to drink a lot of liquids?		
Do you feel that you get colds or infections more frequently than most people you know?		
Are you tired most of the time?		
Do you suffer from infertility or, for women, have symptoms of polycystic ovarian syndrome (irregular cycles, facial hair, and acne)?		
For men: Do you suffer from impotence or erectile dysfunction?		
Do you have jock itch, vaginal yeast infections, anal itching, toenail fungus, dry scaly patches on your skin, or other symptoms of chronic fungal infections?		
Subtotal		

Next, score *three points* for each of the following questions you answer "yes" to.

Comprehensive Diabesity Quiz, Part II	YES	NO
Is your BMI higher than 30?		
Is your waist-to-height ratio greater than 49 if you are a woman or greater than 53 if you are a man?		
Have you been diagnosed with type 2 diabetes, pre-diabetes, or gestational diabetes?		
Has anyone in your family had diabetes, hypoglycemia, or alcoholism?		
Are you of nonwhite ancestry (African, Asian, Native American, Hispanic, Pacific Islander, Indian, Middle Eastern)?		
Do you have high blood pressure?		

continues on next page

Comprehensive Diabesity Quiz, Part II (*continued*)	YES	NO
Have you had a heart attack, angina, transient ischemic attack, or stroke?		
Do you have cataracts or have you ever had retinopathy (eye damage from diabetes)?		
Do you have levels of triglycerides over 100 mg/dl or HDL (good) cholesterol levels less than 50 mg/dl, or blood glucose over 100 mg/dl?		
Do you have kidney damage or protein in your urine?		
Do you have a loss of sensation in your feet or legs?		
Subtotal		
GRAND TOTAL (add subtotals together)		

SCORING KEY

Once you have completed the quiz, determine how severe your condition is and whether you should go on the Basic or Advanced Plan by using this scoring key:

SCORE	SEVERITY	BASIC OR ADVANCED PLAN
1–7	Mild Diabesity	Basic Plan
8+	Moderate to Severe Diabesity	Advanced Plan

Get Tested for Diabesity

You may want to get your blood tested to learn more about your diabesity. Blood tests are useful in helping you identify whether you have diabesity, and how severe it is, and in tracking your progress over time. Ninety percent of people with diabesity are not diagnosed. Testing helps you confirm the diagnosis. Some labs let you order tests on yourself, or you can ask your doctor for these tests. Visit bloodsugarsolution.com/

get-tested-for-diabesity to learn what tests you should have, and download the free guide *How to Work with Your Doctor to Get What You Need.*

HOW DO I REVERSE MY DIABESITY?

Now that you know whether you have basic or advanced diabesity, you can get started. The recipes and meal ideas in this book will start you on a path to healing faster than you can say "sugar." Not only will you lose weight and reduce the need for medication and insulin, but you will have more energy, be in a better mood, and even have a stronger sex drive. And many other chronic symptoms and diseases might just go away—because you are putting healing medicine (food) in your system in ways that turn all the right dials on your biology and give you an immediate biological upgrade.

Food Is Medicine: A Calorie Is Not a Calorie!

The Blood Sugar Solution and this cookbook are based on one very simple but powerful principle: *food is medicine.* Whole, real, fresh food has been proven to be the most powerful drug on the planet, improving the expression of thousands of genes, balancing dozens of hormones, optimizing the function of tens of thousands of protein networks. It can upgrade your biological software. It works faster, better, and cheaper than any other drug and has no side effects. If applied in the right way, it has the power to transform your biology and health—not in months or years, but in days or weeks.

WHAT IS THE DIFFERENCE BETWEEN THE BASIC PLAN AND THE ADVANCED PLAN?

If you took the comprehensive quiz you know whether you need the Basic or Advanced Plan for the Blood Sugar Solution. The Basic Plan is for people who have mild diabesity or who would simply like to prevent it. If you are on the Basic Plan, then a slightly higher carbohydrate load is permitted, as long as your body tolerates it. Small amounts of gluten-free whole grains and nutrient-dense starches, such as sweet potato and squash, as well as a moderate intake of fruit, are acceptable on this plan. But the foundation should be high-quality protein, fats, and nonstarchy vegetables (see Chapter 2 for a list of acceptable foods). If you reach the end of the program and still want better results, try the Advanced Plan for six weeks.

If you qualify for the Advanced Plan, you can reverse diabesity by adhering to a very low-glycemic diet. You can reboot your metabolism, but you have to be much more focused and committed. Many of my diabetic patients get off insulin and medication and reverse diabetes using this approach. The results are worth it. Even in six weeks you can see a profound difference. The diet is essentially one that our hunter-gatherer ancestors ate—protein and plants. Proteins include grass-fed meats or free-range chicken, low-mercury fish, omega-3 eggs, and nuts and seeds. A small amount of beans may be tolerated by some but can raise blood sugar in others. Notice what happens to you. Grains are gone! The only fruit allowed is berries—and only a small amount (½ cup). And vegetables must be low in starch—for example, cruciferous vegetables, green beans, all manner of crunchy vegetables, and sea vegetables, but no starchy veggies like winter squash, potatoes, or sweet potatoes.

Some of you might be interested in trying the recipes even if you are not on the program. By all means—please do! Notice how you feel when you eat whole, real, metabolism-boosting and -balancing foods. Explore how to cook with whole foods. Are you sensitive to gluten and/or dairy and want new allergen-free recipes to add to your mix? Have you heard how people's lives have been transformed when they get rid of junk and sugar from their diet? *The Blood Sugar Solution Cookbook* will help you discover food that inspires you, delights you, stimulates you, and invigorates you. Food to live by and food to heal by!

I asked my community to help create this cookbook. I combined their contributions with my own favorite recipes. I carefully read and tested each recipe and worked with my nutrition team to ensure that each ingredient fits within the guidelines of the Blood Sugar Solution. I have made many of these recipes with my friends and family and, I promise, you will not be disappointed.

One last note. Let this cookbook bring out the inner nutritionist and chef in you. While following recipes is often helpful, fun, and nonstressful, you don't need recipes in order to eat well. Often we forget how pleasurable it is to tune into our senses and use our intuition to literally play with our food. Traditional cultures didn't rely on cookbooks—they used the most abundant foods in season to create nutritious meals that allowed our species to evolve and thrive. And, yes, while recipes can be a way to form community and pass on timeless rituals from one generation to the next, they can also help you create new rituals that represent your own beliefs, values, and tastes. Challenge yourself to create your own recipes and rituals for your family. Start your own cooking revolution!

2

Preparing for the Blood Sugar Solution

STEP 1: PREPARE YOUR KITCHEN

Have you noticed that people love to gather in the kitchen? It is the place for nourishment and receiving life's comforts. Good conversation, bonding with friends and family, and creating meals to sustain us all take root here. The sad thing about today's fast-paced lifestyle is that it can be really difficult to slow down and spend time in this sacred space. Worse, it can be easier to grab convenient junk food if that's what's hanging around the home. These disease-creating foods are a sure obstacle to your success with the Blood Sugar Solution way of life. We have hundreds of genes that protect us from starvation, but very few that protect us from overeating. What we need is a lifestyle that makes cooking healthy, easy, and fun. It is time to get back to our roots and take back our kitchens!

When I was a boy, my mother told me, "If you can read, you can cook." You don't have to be Julia Child or Mario Batali. You can learn to create nourishing, delicious, and healthy meals quickly and inexpensively without enrolling in cooking school. Does this seem difficult to accomplish while living a full life with a never-ending schedule? You might be surprised to find it's not. It just takes a little practice and planning.

If you are reluctant to cook or think you don't have the time, these recipes might just save you from yourself. Most Americans spend more time watching cooking on television than actually cooking! Look carefully at your days, at where you invest your time and energy, and you just might find that investing your time in preparing real food delivers higher dividends in health, pleasure, and connection to others.

Get Your Essential Kitchen Tools

Would you start any journey without the necessary equipment? Of course not! Following is a list of the tools you need for the care and feeding of a human being—*you,* and your friends and family. Give yourself permission to invest in high-quality kitchen tools that will last a lifetime. A well-stocked kitchen makes cooking simple, fast, and fun. I suggest you try to have most of these in your kitchen:

- a set of good-quality knives
- 2 wooden cutting boards—one for animal products, another for fruits and vegetables
- an 8-inch and a 12-inch nonstick (non-Teflon) sauté pan, preferably Calphalon or All-Clad
- an 8-quart stockpot
- a 2-quart and a 4-quart saucepan with lids
- an 11-inch-square nonstick (non-Teflon) stovetop griddle
- a Dutch oven
- a grill pan
- 3 or 4 cookie or baking sheets
- a food processor
- a blender
- an immersion blender
- an instant-read chef's thermometer
- a can opener
- a coffee grinder for flaxseed and spices
- wire whisks
- spring tongs
- a fish spatula
- rubber spatulas
- assorted measuring cups, metal for dry ingredients and glass for liquids
- a lemon/citrus reamer

- microplane graters in assorted sizes
- a food mill
- natural parchment paper and foil
- glass storage containers with lids
- a tea ball
- a timer

For more ideas and to see my favorite supplies, go to bloodsugar-solution.com/healthy-living-resources/.

Have Fun in the Kitchen

Some people hate being in the kitchen. They don't like to cook. They find chopping vegetables boring. They feel that standing over a stove sautéing fish is as interesting as watching a pot of water boil. They just don't enjoy the time they spend in the kitchen. But cooking is an essential life survival skill that we should all cultivate and pass on to our children. Personally, I love being in the kitchen. I enjoy spending my time looking for and preparing wholesome, delicious foods that allow me and my family to thrive.

The kitchen can become a happy, social, fun place to be. Perhaps one of the differences between people who love the kitchen and people who hate it is the kind of environment they create. Here are some simple, wonderful tips to make cooking easier and more enjoyable.

- **Play music.** OK, I'll admit it. Standing there chopping vegetables and fresh herbs in silence isn't always the most entertaining job in the world. But it doesn't have to be boring! Play music on the radio, a CD player, or your iPod while you prepare and cook your food. Chop to the music. Get some veggies ready for the week, make a ready-to-eat salad, cook up some grains, and even prepare a recipe or two that you can have on hand for a busy weeknight meal—all to the sounds of your favorite tunes.
- **Get the family involved.** Even if your spouse doesn't cook, you can still lure him or her into the kitchen to chat with you while you

cook. Even better, get your kids involved in the kitchen. It's a great way to connect with them and make the experience more fun while educating them about real, whole foods. This can help counter some of the messages they are getting from the media.

- **Open up the kitchen.** Laboring away under fluorescent lights in some corner of your house chopping vegetables for an hour is a sure way to get sick of being in the kitchen. As much as possible, open up your kitchen. Open doors and windows. Invest in good lighting. Decorate. Bring in bar stools or a small table. Make the kitchen a place you and your family want to be.
- **Try new things.** One surefire way to get bored in the kitchen is by preparing the same things over and over. Try new recipes. Experiment with new cooking techniques. Use *The Blood Sugar Solution Cookbook* to help you enjoy your time in the kitchen!
- **Be patient, not perfect.** With practice, you will become comfortable in the kitchen.
- **Make one day a week a food prep day.** Gather your recipes, write your shopping lists, go to the store (preferably after a meal or a small snack), and buy only what's on your list.
- **Try not to be intimidated by recipes.** Simply read them from start to finish and visualize the process. If something doesn't make sense or you can't picture it, reread it until you are ready. Then begin cooking! And follow along step by step. Remember: if you can read, you can cook.
- **Multitask.** I don't usually advocate multitasking—except in the kitchen. While you cook some quinoa on the stove, why not chop some vegetables for a stew or salad?
- **Double or triple your recipes and freeze some for later use.** You will be happy when life gets busy and you realize you have access to a homemade meal.

I hope the suggestions in this section offer you insight about how to make your time in the kitchen enjoyable and efficient.

Detox Your Kitchen

Set aside an hour or so to investigate all possible disease-creating suspects in your pantry and send them off to the dump. If it is not a real, whole food, toss it. It has no place in your Blood Sugar Solution kitchen. Not sure how to tell the good from the bad? Read on.

10 RULES FOR EATING SAFELY FOR LIFE (AND WHAT TO REMOVE FROM YOUR KITCHEN)

Follow these rules for getting healthy, losing weight, and feeling great:

1. **Focus on foods without labels—that is, foods that don't come in a box, bag, or can.** There are some perfectly good packaged foods out there, like sardines or roasted red peppers, but you must learn to read labels in order to buy wisely. Look carefully at the ingredient list and the nutrition facts. The most abundant ingredient is listed first and the others are listed in descending order by weight. Be conscious, too, of ingredients that may not be on the list; some ingredients may be exempt from labels. This is often true if the food is in a very small package, if it has been prepared in the store, or if it was made by a small manufacturer. Stay clear of these foods.

2. **If a food has a label, it should have fewer than five ingredients.** If it has more than five ingredients, throw it out. Also, beware of food with health claims on the label. These foods are usually bad for you—"sports beverages" or "energy bars," for example.

3. **If sugar by any name is on the label (including organic cane juice, honey, agave nectar, maple syrup, cane syrup, or molasses), throw it out.** There may be up to 33 teaspoons of sugar—often high-fructose corn syrup—in the average bottle of ketchup. And even though refined grains and flour are not technically sugar, they act just like sugar in the body. If you have diabesity, you can't easily

handle any flour, even whole-grain. Throw it out. And stay away from white rice.

4. **Throw out any food with high-fructose corn syrup on the label.** This super-sweet liquid sugar is quickly absorbed, goes right to your liver, and kicks fat production into high gear. Some high-fructose corn syrup also contains mercury as a by-product of the manufacturing process. Many liquid calories, such as sodas, juices, and sports drinks, contain this metabolic poison. It always signals low-quality or processed food.

5. **Throw out any food with the word "hydrogenated" on the label.** This signals trans fats, which are dangerous vegetable oils converted through a chemical process into margarine or shortening that block our metabolism, create inflammation, and cause diabetes.

6. **Throw out any highly refined cooking oils such as corn and soy.** Avoid these refined toxic fats and any foods fried in them.

7. **Throw out any food with ingredients you can't recognize or pronounce, or that are in Latin.**

8. **Throw out any food with preservatives, additives, coloring or dyes, "natural flavorings," or flavor enhancers such as MSG** (monosodium glutamate). MSG is a brain toxin that causes compulsive overeating.

9. **Throw out food with artificial sweeteners of all kinds** (aspartame, NutraSweet, Splenda, sucralose, and sugar alcohols— any word that ends with "ol," like xylitol or sorbitol). They make you hungry, lower your metabolism, create gas, and store belly fat.

10. **Throw out anything that didn't come from the earth.** As Michael Pollan says, if it was grown on a plant, not made in a plant, then you can keep it in your kitchen. If it is something your great-grandmother wouldn't recognize as food (like a Lunchable or Go-Gurt), throw it out. Stay away from "foodlike substances."

That's it—just 10 goof-proof rules for staying healthy for life. These will keep you out of trouble and automatically lead you to a real, whole-foods diet. When you make these simple choices, not only will you improve your health and the health of your family, you will also create a shift in demand in the marketplace. You will help America take back its health. You vote three times a day with your fork, and this impacts our collective health, how we grow our food, our energy consumption, climate change, and environmental degradation. You have more power than you think. Use it!

STEP 2: SHOP

Stock Your Pantry

The key to success in the kitchen is to have the right ingredients on hand when the inspiration hits you. I make sure to stock my kitchen well, so that I can always whip up a meal from whatever's in my cupboard and fridge. These are the staples everyone should have to make delicious and spontaneous meals and create great health.

LEGUMES

The legume family includes a wide variety of beans, all of which serve as a great source of protein. Look for these beans at your supermarket:

adzuki beans	Great Northern beans
black beans	kidney beans
black-eyed peas	lentils
butter beans/baby lima beans	mung beans
cannellini beans	navy beans
chickpeas/garbanzo beans	pinto beans
fava beans/broad beans	split peas

When buying canned beans, seek out BPA-free cans. BPA, or bisphenol A, is used in plastics and the lining of cans, and causes insulin resistance, weight gain, and diabetes. Or, better yet, cook with dried beans from the bulk section of your local market. The following instructions show you how to make the tastiest and most easily digested beans.

Soaking dried beans: Large beans need to be soaked in filtered water for 8 to 12 hours before cooking. While small beans and lentils can be cooked without soaking, you can decrease the cooking time and improve digestibility if you soak them for a couple of hours. Discard the soaking water before cooking.

Using kombu: Kombu, or dried kelp, is rich in minerals, trace elements, and vitamins. Cooking beans with a small piece of this nutritious sea vegetable increases flavor and nutrition while also decreasing the amount of time they need to cook. And this special seaweed reduces flatulence caused by improperly prepared beans. It is really easy to use kombu; all you need is one 1-inch piece per cup of beans.

Cooking beans: Drain the soaked beans and place them in a pot, cover with filtered water, and bring to a boil. If you see a film of foam form over the top of your beans, simply skim it off with a spoon — this will help decrease gas. Toss in your kombu, reduce the heat to a simmer, and cover the pot for the remainder of the cooking time. When the beans are tender, drain any remaining water and discard the kombu. The cooking time for beans varies, depending on their size:

BEANS (1 CUP DRIED)	WATER	COOKING TIME
adzuki beans, soaked	3 cups	45–60 minutes
other large beans (black, navy, pinto, etc.), soaked	3–4 cups	1 ½–2 hours
soybeans, soaked	4 cups	2–3 hours
black-eyed peas, unsoaked	3 cups	30–45 minutes
brown or green lentils, unsoaked	3 cups	45 minutes
red lentils, unsoaked	3 cups	15–30 minutes
green or yellow split peas, unsoaked	3–4 cups	50–60 minutes

The legume family also includes soybeans and products made from soybeans. These, when used in the traditional forms noted opposite, are a good source of protein and minerals:

edamame	soybeans
miso	tempeh
natto	tofu

Make sure all beans and soy products are organic and non-GMO (genetically modified organisms, which have been proven to cause cancer and other adverse health effects).

MY FAVORITE SOURCES FOR LEGUMES:

Eden Foods	WestSoy
Soy Dream	WhiteWave
Westbrae Natural	WholeSoy & Co.

SEAFOOD

Whenever possible, choose wild over farmed fish. For guidelines on low-mercury fish, visit nrdc.org/health/effects/mercury/walletcard.pdf to download a wallet card you can carry with you for reference when you are shopping. Choose from these low-mercury fish:

anchovy	mackerel/chub mackerel
butterfish	(North Atlantic)
catfish	mullet
clam	oyster
crab (domestic)	perch (ocean)
crawfish/crayfish	plaice
croaker (Atlantic)	pollock
flounder*	salmon (canned or fresh)
haddock (Atlantic)*	sardine
hake	scallop*
herring	shad (American)

---

* These fish may be in danger because of depleted stocks or nonsustainable harvesting practices. See www.montereybayaquarium.org/cr/cr_seafoodwatch/download.aspx.

shrimp*
sole (Pacific)
squid/calamari
tilapia

trout (freshwater)
whitefish
whiting

MY FAVORITE SOURCES FOR SAFE FISH:

CleanFish
Crown Prince Natural
EcoFish

SeaBear
Vital Choice

OMEGA-3 EGGS

Choose organic eggs from grass-fed, hormone- and antibiotic-free chickens. If possible, buy locally sourced eggs.

MY FAVORITE SOURCES FOR HIGH-QUALITY EGGS:

Organic Valley
Pete & Gerry's Organics

POULTRY

Choose grass-fed, organic, hormone- and antibiotic-free, and, if possible, locally sourced poultry. It is a good source of lean protein. Focus on these types of poultry:

boneless, skinless chicken breasts
ground chicken or turkey
turkey or turkey breasts

MY FAVORITE SOURCES FOR HIGH-QUALITY POULTRY:

Bell & Evans
local farmer's markets

---

* These fish may be in danger because of depleted stocks or nonsustainable harvesting practices. See www.montereybayaquarium.org/cr/cr_seafoodwatch/download.aspx.

Murray's Chicken
Plainville Farms
Whole Foods Market

MEAT

Select grass-fed, organic, hormone- and antibiotic-free, and, if possible, locally sourced meat. Look for lean beef, lean lamb, and bison (buffalo) meat.

MY FAVORITE SOURCES FOR HIGH-QUALITY MEAT:
community supported agriculture (CSA's)
Eatwild
local farms or farmer's markets
Whole Foods Market

See ewg.org/meateatersguide for a guide to eating meat that is both good for you and good for the planet. Meat that is sustainably raised, grass-fed, and free of hormones and antibiotics lessens the impact on the environment and the effects on climate change—and it's better for your body!

FRESH VEGETABLES AND FRUITS

Choose organic, seasonal, and local produce whenever possible. Sometimes organic vegetables and fruits are best purchased frozen if they are not in season—for example, berries in the winter months. While organic produce tends to be nutritionally superior to its conventionally grown counterparts, if you need to prioritize, the Environmental Working Group has prepared lists of the "Clean Fifteen" and the "Dirty Dozen" (visit ewg.org/foodnews for updated lists and to download a pocket guide or smart phone app).

CLEAN FIFTEEN: LOWEST IN PESTICIDES—OKAY TO BUY
CONVENTIONAL (in order from least to more toxic):
onions   avocado
sweet corn   cabbage
pineapple   sweet peas

asparagus

mangoes

eggplant

kiwi

cantaloupe (domestic)

sweet potatoes

grapefruit

watermelon

mushrooms

DIRTY DOZEN: HIGHEST IN PESTICIDES—BUY ORGANIC (in order of most to least pesticide used):

apples

celery

sweet bell peppers

peaches

strawberries

nectarines (imported)

grapes

spinach

lettuce

cucumbers

blueberries (domestic)

potatoes

kale and other greens

green beans

Think of your grocery store as your pharmacy—it is where you will find the world's most powerful medicines. As you wander through the produce aisles, pick out Mother Nature's best drugs:

- red, yellow, and orange fruits and vegetables: bell peppers, carrots, chile peppers, pumpkins, raspberries, strawberries, sweet potatoes/ yams, tomatoes, turnips, winter squash
- dark green leafy vegetables: arugula, beet greens, collard greens, dandelion greens, kale, lettuce, mustard greens, spinach, Swiss chard
- dark blue, purple, or red fruits and vegetables: beets, blackberries, blueberries, cherries, eggplant, plums, radicchio, radishes, red cabbage, red onions
- cruciferous vegetables: bok choy, broccoli, broccoli sprouts, Brussels sprouts, cabbage, cauliflower, Chinese broccoli, collards, kale, kohlrabi, turnips
- allium vegetables: garlic, leeks, onions, scallions, shallots
- citrus fruits: lemons, limes
- sea vegetables: arame, dulse, hijiki, kombu
- low-glycemic fruits and vegetables: apples, asparagus, avocados, celery, green beans, pears, snap peas, snow peas, stone fruit (apricots, nectarines, peaches, and plums), zucchini

- konjac (the bulb of a Japanese plant that is all fiber, has no calories, and is used to make shirataki noodles)

MY FAVORITE SOURCES FOR ORGANIC PRODUCE:

Cascadian Farm	Maine Coast Sea Vegetables
Earthbound Farm	Miracle Noodle
local farmer's markets and CSA's	Stahlbush Island Farms

WHOLE GRAINS

For those on the Basic Plan, gluten-free, low-glycemic grains in moderate portions (½ cup daily) can be a great source of vitamins, minerals, and fiber. Avoid these if you're on the Advanced Plan.

amaranth	millet
brown and black rice	quinoa
buckwheat/kasha	teff

MY FAVORITE SOURCES FOR GLUTEN-FREE GRAINS:

Arrowhead Mills	Lundberg Family Farms
Hodgson Mill	Shiloh Farms

"FLOURS"

Nut meal is a great alternative to grain-based flours, which can be very high-glycemic. By choosing to bake and cook with these alternatives, you boost your intake of restorative fiber and minerals while avoiding a nasty blood-sugar-spiking glycemic load.

almond meal
coconut flour

MY FAVORITE SOURCE FOR HIGH-QUALITY FLOUR ALTERNATIVES:
Bob's Red Mill

NUTS AND SEEDS

Choose raw or sprouted nuts and seeds, and organic if possible. You can always lightly roast or toast nuts at home. This allows you to control the temperature and avoid eating rancid and oxidized nuts. Ground nuts and seeds make for wonderful nut butters and healthy oils. You can also use nut "milks" as a healthy alternative to dairy.

almonds	pecans
Brazil nuts	pine nuts
cashews	pistachios
flaxseeds, chia seeds, and hemp seeds	pumpkin seeds, sesame seeds, and sunflower seeds
hazelnuts	walnuts
macadamia nuts	

MY FAVORITE SOURCES FOR HIGH-QUALITY NUTS AND SEEDS:

Artisana	Once Again
Barlean's Organic Oils	Pacific Foods
Eden Foods	Spectrum
MaraNatha	WhiteWave
Omega Nutrition	

HERBS, SPICES, AND SEASONINGS

Choose phytonutrient-rich and flavorful herbs, spices, and seasonings to add depth to your meals. There's no need to mask fresh, whole foods with excess salt or sweeteners when you can add color, flavor, and aroma as well as powerful disease-busting chemicals to all your dishes.

basil (fresh and dried)	cayenne powder
bay leaf (dried)	chili powder
black pepper	chipotle powder
broth or stock	cilantro (fresh)

cinnamon

cooking wines (such as Japanese Mirin)

coriander

cumin

curry powder

dill (fresh and dried)

ginger (fresh and powdered)

jalapeño peppers (fresh)

mustards

parsley (fresh and dried)

red chili paste

rosemary (fresh and dried)

sage (fresh and dried)

sea salt

sriracha

tahini

tamari

thyme (fresh and dried)

tomato sauce and paste

Vegenaise

vinegars

MY FAVORITE SOURCES FOR HIGH-QUALITY SEASONINGS:

Edward & Sons

Flavorganics

Frontier Natural Products Co-Op

Penzeys Spices

Rapunzel

Seeds of Change

The Spice Hunter

HEALTHY FATS AND OILS

Select organic and unrefined whenever possible.

avocados and avocado oil

coconut butter

flaxseed oil

grapeseed oil

olives and extra-virgin olive oil

sesame oil (light or dark)

tahini

walnut oil

MY FAVORITE SOURCES FOR HIGH-QUALITY OILS:

Artisana

Barlean's Organic Oils

Spectrum

MY TOP SUPERFOODS

These superfoods have a high concentration of anti-inflammatory, detoxifying, disease-busting phytochemicals, blood-sugar-balancing fats, and high-quality protein.

SUPER VEGETABLES

- arugula
- beets
- broccoli family (broccoli, Brussels sprouts, cabbage, collards, kale, kohlrabi)
- cilantro
- dandelion greens
- onions
- parsley
- sea vegetables
- shiitake mushrooms
- shirataki noodles (from konjac)
- sprouts (especially broccoli sprouts)
- sweet potatoes
- watercress

SUPER FRUITS

- apples
- avocados
- berries (especially wild, organic blueberries, acai, and goji)
- kiwis
- lemons
- pomegranates

SUPER SPICES AND FOODS

- cacao (raw)
- chiles
- cinnamon
- garlic
- ginger
- green tea/matcha
- miso
- turmeric

SUPER PROTEIN SOURCES

- adzuki beans
- black beans

- edamame
- nuts (especially almonds, Brazil nuts, pine nuts, and walnuts)
- omega-3 eggs
- sardines
- seeds (especially chia, flax, hemp, pumpkin, and sunflower)
- wild salmon (fresh or canned)

SUPER FATS
- extra-virgin coconut butter
- extra-virgin olive oil

LOW-GLYCEMIC VEGETABLES: UNLIMITED REFILLS

There are certain "free foods" that are so low in calories and so nutrient-dense that you can't overeat them. If you want to binge, these are the foods to choose. They should be the bulk of your diet; they should take up 50 percent to 75 percent of your plate at every meal. In fact, you can enjoy these plant foods in unlimited quantities. Keep a list of these with you when you go shopping and make them the new staples of your diet. I often make two or three vegetable dishes every night. Find fun, easy ways to prepare them.

- artichokes
- arugula
- asparagus
- bean sprouts
- beet greens
- bell peppers
- broccoli
- Brussels sprouts
- cabbage
- cauliflower
- celery
- chives
- collard greens
- cucumbers
- dandelion greens
- eggplant
- endive
- garlic
- ginger root
- green beans
- hearts of palm
- jalapeño peppers
- kale
- lettuce
- mushrooms
- mustard greens

- onions
- parsley
- radicchio
- radishes
- shallots
- snap beans
- snow peas
- spinach
- summer squash
- Swiss chard
- tomatoes
- turnip greens
- watercress
- zucchini

Serving Sizes

Size does matter! So does variety and frequency. Follow these guidelines:

- Eat three meals each day with two snacks.
- Each meal can have up to 15 grams of carbohydrates, and each snack can have up to 7.5 grams. If you exercise regularly or increase your exercise routine while on this program, you can slowly begin to increase these amounts. But have no more than 30 grams of carbohydrates at a meal unless they come from low-glycemic vegetables such as broccoli, green beans, asparagus, salad greens, etc.
- As your insulin sensitivity improves, you can increase your consumption of natural carbohydrates to 30 to 50 grams per meal. Choose nonstarchy vegetables, whole grains, legumes, and lower-glycemic fruit such as blueberries, raspberries, apples, and pears. You should eliminate refined carbohydrates and sugars for the first six weeks on the program, then you can have an occasional small treat once a week if it doesn't trigger sugar or carb bingeing.

The following serving sizes are based on cooked servings unless otherwise noted; each serving contains 15 grams of carbohydrates. In general, sweet potatoes, beans, lentils, and squash have a glycemic index of around 50—medium-burning but great in the right portion size (½ sweet potato or ½ cup beans, lentils, or cooked squash). These don't include every item you might eat, but are a sampling to get a sense of correct portion size. It is often smaller than we think.

The Glycemic Index and Glycemic Load

Not all foods with the same number of grams of carbohydrate raise your blood sugar in the same way. Some, especially those low in fiber, cause a rapid spike in blood sugar levels. Others lead to a slow, sustained rise. Using the glycemic index and glycemic load is a way to quantify these differences in foods.

What is the GI?

You may have heard about the **glycemic index (GI)**. It measures how 50 grams of carbohydrates from a specific food raises your blood sugar levels compared to 50 grams of glucose (a pure simple sugar). The index is measured on a scale of 0 to 100, with glucose having a value of 100. **Higher numbers mean a food causes a sharper rise in blood sugar.**

> High GI: 70 and up
> Medium GI: 56–69
> Low GI: 55 and under

Why does it matter?

Having a general idea of a food's glycemic index helps you put together meals and snacks that provide a slow, sustained rise in your blood sugar for lasting energy. This may help you:

- feel fuller or more satisfied for a longer period of time to help prevent cravings.
- help maintain or obtain an ideal weight.
- choose unprocessed, high fiber carbohydrates.

What are its limits?

The glycemic index can't be used alone to plan a healthy diet. It won't tell you:

- whether a food is rich in nutrients — so keep choosing whole foods.

continues on next page

- how different cooking methods, like mashing, will affect a given GI.
- the GI for many foods that haven't been tested yet.

The glycemic index also won't tell you the **glycemic load (GL), which is the impact a chosen serving of food has on your blood sugar.** Glycemic load depends on a food, serving size, total carbohydrate grams, and fiber. For example, kiwis have a medium glycemic index (58), but a serving of just one kiwi is considered low GL (5). The GL numbers are classified on the following scale:

High GL: 20 or more
Medium GL: 11–19
Low GL: 0–10

This means that when you consume larger portions, or add a higher-glycemic food on the side, it raises the overall glycemic load of your meal. On the other hand, pairing a carb-containing food with healthy fats or protein helps you reduce the overall glycemic load of your meal or snack. Try combinations like these to balance your blood sugar:

brown rice or carrots with roasted turkey
whole-grain crackers with a hard-boiled egg
freshly sliced apple with almond butter

It's also important to realize that certain foods, such as agave nectar, contain more of the sugar *fructose*. These foods appear lower on the glycemic index because the scale is based on blood *glucose* (a different type of sugar). Continue to moderate your intake of foods high in fructose because research suggests that excess consumption of the sugar promotes fat storage.

How can I use it?

You can calculate the glycemic load for any food, but if you combine good-quality protein, good fats, and low-glycemic carbs, you will create low-glycemic meals. Adding fiber, protein, or fat to any carbohydrate will also lower the glycemic load of the meal.

STARCHY VEGETABLES

Food Item	Serving	Food Item	Serving
artichokes	1	parsnips	⅔ cup
beets	1 cup	potatoes (baked)	½ medium
burdock (raw)	½ medium	pumpkin	1 cup
carrots	1 cup	sweet potatoes/yams (baked)	½ medium
corn	½ cup	turnips	½ cup
green peas	½ cup	winter squash	½ cup
Jerusalem artichokes/ sunchokes	½ cup		

LEGUMES

Food Item	Serving	Food Item	Serving
adzuki beans	¼ cup	kidney beans	⅓ cup
black beans	⅓ cup	lentils	⅓ cup
black-eyed peas	½ cup	mung beans	⅓ cup
broad beans	½ cup	navy or pinto beans	⅓ cup
chickpeas	⅓ cup	split peas	⅓ cup
French lentils	⅓ cup		

GRAINS

Food Item	Serving	Food Item	Serving
brown rice	⅓ cup	popcorn (popped)	2½ cups
buckwheat/kasha	⅓ cup	quinoa	⅓ cup
millet	⅓ cup	teff	⅓ cup
polenta	⅓ cup		

WHOLE-GRAIN FLOUR AND MEAL

Food Item	Serving	Food Item	Serving
amaranth flour	2 tbsp	brown rice flour	2 tbsp
arrowroot flour	2 tbsp	buckwheat flour	3½ tbsp

FRUIT (RAW, UNLESS OTHERWISE NOTED)

Food Item	Serving	Food Item	Serving
apples (fresh)	1 small	applesauce (unsweetened)	¾ cup
apples (dried)	3 rings	apricots (fresh)	2 medium

FRUIT (RAW, UNLESS OTHERWISE NOTED, cont'd)

Food Item	Serving	Food Item	Serving
apricots (dried)	7 halves	oranges	1 medium
avocados	½ medium	peaches	1 medium
berries	¾ cup	pears	½ large
cherries	1 cup	plums	2 medium
currants (dried)	2 tbsp	prunes/dried plums	3 medium
dates (dried)	2 medium	raisins	2 tbsp
figs (dried)	1 medium	strawberries	1½ cups
grapefruit	½ large	tangerines	2 small
kiwis	1 large	tomatoes (fresh)	1 medium
mangoes	½ medium	tomatoes (sun-dried)	2 tbsp
nectarines	1 medium		

PROTEIN

Food Item	Serving
fish	4 ounces (size of your palm)
chicken	4 ounces
meat	4 ounces
nuts and seeds	3 tbsp (small handful)
tofu and tempeh	4 ounces

CRACKERS

These are less wholesome carbohydrate options than those given above, but they are convenient; whole grains are always a better option. I recommend gluten-free, seed-based crackers like Mary's Gone Crackers rather than high-glycemic rice cakes or crackers.

Food Item	Serving
rice cakes	2
rice crackers	4
flax or seed crackers	4

Eat Well for Less

By now some of you might be wondering how to make this work on your budget. Eating well can be an eye-opening experience when you learn a few simple tricks. Try the following:

- Because cheap food is inexpensive due to subsidization, it might seem that you have to buy junk food in order to stay within your budget. Track all of your expenses for one week and observe how much of what you spend your money on contributes to achieving your health goals. If you notice certain items do not serve your ultimate health goals, then perhaps this is a good place to start rearranging your spending habits. For example, one cup of Starbucks at $4 a day adds up to $1,460 a year. Make your own coffee!
- Reorganize your budget and priorities, and you might create more funding for good food. For example, can you pack your lunch, saving money for high-quality food?
- Money represents your life energy. Every dollar you make you pay for with time. How you spend your money reflects how you spend your time. Think about how you can make more conscious choices about the way you spend your money.
- Make choices that give you more resources: Choose three things to change that can give you more time or money and record them in your journal. Reflect on how your life and health change as you go through the six weeks of the program.
- Shop at neighborhood stores or discount stores like Trader Joe's or shopping clubs like Costco.
- Develop a repertoire of cheap, healthy, easy-to-prepare meals that decrease stress, time, and cost.
- Grow your own veggies or herbs in a windowsill pot, backyard garden, or community plot.

Read Labels When You Really Must Buy Processed Foods

Organic and whole foods are now available in packages, cans, and boxes. They tend to be found in natural foods stores or the health food section of your regular grocery store.

Even if a particular food item has ingredients you are familiar with, you may want to avoid certain ingredients in processed or manufactured foods. For example, you will want to be careful not to inadvertently include foods in your diet that aren't allowed on the program.

Labels list the ingredients and some of the nutrition information. Be sure to read all food labels carefully as you shop for the ingredients you will use while on the program. This will help you adhere to the guidelines of the Blood Sugar Solution as closely as possible.

Here are things to be aware of:

- **Beware of health claims on the label.** Food packaging and labels represent marketing at its cleverest. Look for high-quality ingredients and don't be fooled by exaggerated claims. My usual rule is that if it has a health claim, it is probably not good for you.
- **Watch for where an ingredient appears on the list.** If the real food is at the end of the list and the sugars or salts are at the beginning, beware. The most abundant ingredient is listed first, and the others are listed in descending order by weight.
- **Beware of ingredients in foods that are not labeled.** Foods in very small packages, foods prepared in the store, and foods made by small manufacturers are exempt from labels.
- **Look for additives or problem ingredients.** If a food contains high-fructose corn syrup, hydrogenated oils, or partially hydrogenated oils, put it back on the shelf. Also look out for sulfites, nitrites, and any funny-sounding preservatives or fillers that don't seem familiar or safe to you. If you can't recognize or pronounce the ingredient, it is probably not fit for human consumption.

- **Look for hidden sources of gluten and dairy.** Gluten can be lurking in soba noodles, tamari, miso, seasonings, and broth, so look for a gluten-free option. Dairy can be found in mayonnaise, chocolate, and "natural" flavors and anything that has casein (look for it on the food ingredient list). Beware!

- **Look for sneaky pseudo-names for sugar.** Sugar comes in many forms and textures. Honey, syrup, sugar cane crystals, sugar alcohols (xylitol, maltitol, etc.), powders, fruit juices, dried fruit, natural sugars, artificial sweeteners, refined sugars, concentrated, dehydrated, malted, fermented sugars, molasses, sorghum, and liquid sweeteners are all sugar.

- **Would your great-grandmother have served this food?** Finally, before you analyze the numbers, ask yourself whether this food could have been served at your great-grandmother's table. If not, beware.

Understanding the Nutrition Label: Think Low GL and High PI

Glycemic load (GL) is a measure of how quickly a food enters your bloodstream. A low-GL diet leads to better health and is the only diet that has been proven to work for long-term weight loss. In fact, eating a low-GL diet can speed up your metabolism by about 300 calories a day—the equivalent of running for one hour a day.

Phytonutrient index (PI) refers to the amount of colorful plant pigments and compounds in a food that help prevent disease and promote health. A high PI also leads to better health. Here are a few tips to help you maintain a low GL and a high PI:

- **Look at the serving size and determine whether this is your "typical" portion,** as labels can be deceiving. A package or bottle might say that it contains 2 or 3 servings, but we have gotten used to eating the whole thing in one sitting. We often eat more than we actually need, especially when it comes to grains. Your goal is to limit grains and legumes to ⅓ to ½ cup regardless of what the box says. Afraid this won't be enough? Fill half your plate with fiber-rich nonstarchy vegetables.

- **Are the calories high GL or low GL?** The total amount of carbohydrates on your plate is less important than where they come from. If they are found in foods with a low GL and high PI, they will have a very different impact on your appetite and weight than foods that are quickly absorbed and have few nutrients and fiber. How do you know which foods have a low GL and high PI? Simple. Choose whole, nonstarchy plant foods, and you can't lose. See pages 33–34 for a list of low-GL vegetables. You get unlimited refills on these.

- **Start with fiber.** Fiber is one of the main factors that determine the all-important GL, and it can also give you a clue about the phytonutrient index. Look for at least 4 grams of fiber per serving. Better yet, by avoiding packaged, processed convenience foods, you will ensure that your diet is full of fiber.

- **Look at total carbohydrates.** Remember that it's the type of carbs that matters most. If they are from whole-plant foods that contain plenty of fiber or have a low GL, their effect is very different from carbs in foods without fiber. The same amount of carbohydrates from a can of beans affects the body very differently than those from a can of cola.

- **Where are the good fats?** Monounsaturated and omega-3 polyunsaturated fats should dominate this category, with minimal amounts of saturated fat (less than 5 grams) and zero trans fats. Although the mention of trans fats has been required on food labels since 2006, small amounts of trans fats are still permitted in packaged foods without being indicated, as long as the food contains less than 0.5 grams of trans fats per serving. That means that if you eat that food frequently or eat more than one serving you may inadvertently get a load of trans fats. Therefore, look carefully at the ingredients list, even if the label says "zero trans fats." Look for the words "hydrogenated" or "partially hydrogenated." If you see those words, put the item back on the shelf.

What Do the "Nutrition Facts" Mean?

Nutrition facts are merely a guide to help you sort out the healthy from the unhealthy foods. The numbers don't mean as much as what's in the food itself, so focus on *quality over quantity*. However, you can use labels to your advantage if you know what to look for. Let's look at what is most relevant to your goal of keeping your blood sugar balanced.

Keep in mind the following when on the Blood Sugar Solution program:

- **Cholesterol.** Worried about the cholesterol in your omega-3 eggs? Your liver makes more cholesterol in an hour than you could ever eat in a day. More cholesterol is produced in the body from eating sugar than from eating fat. There is little correlation between dietary cholesterol and blood cholesterol, and little reason to worry about this number on food labels. Surprising but true.
- **Protein.** Protein is your secret weapon to success on this program because it reduces insulin spikes and provides you with fuel to sustain energy throughout your day. Opt for high-biological-value protein sources such as lean fish, organic poultry, omega-3 eggs, nuts, and fiber-rich legumes. Remember that diversity is the key to nutrition, so eat from a variety of whole foods to meet your protein needs.
- **Sodium.** Most packaged foods have sodium added to give them flavor, but fresh foods don't need much salt to taste fabulous. When you eat whole foods, you naturally get the right amount of sodium your body needs. By following my program, you will easily cut down on and normalize your sodium intake. Play around with adding real flavor to your meals by using tasty spices such as curry, chile peppers, rosemary, sage, and cinnamon. The less salt you add, the less you will want, as your taste buds adapt to new eating habits.
- **Other nutrients.** Sometimes junk foods are fortified with nutrients to enhance their nutrition appeal. For example, B vitamins are added to foods to "enrich" them. But that is only because they are so impoverished in the first place. Do you really think Vitamin Water is anything other than a cleverly disguised sugar drink?

STEP 3: GET READY

How to Cook with a Busy Schedule

One of the questions I am most frequently asked by people who are interested in trying out the Blood Sugar Solution program is: How do I make this plan work on my busy schedule?

Trust me when I say that I know what it's like to be busy. I'm a practicing physician who travels internationally giving presentations and seminars. I write books. I have a family of my own. I'm a busy person just like you. Yet I eat according to the principles outlined in *The Blood Sugar Solution* and cook recipes out of this cookbook or similar ones all the time (well, almost!). How do I manage to do that?

It comes down to one word: planning. If you're anywhere near as busy as I am and you want to make the program work for you, you are going to have to learn to do some things in advance.

I know this may seem like a lot to do when you already have a busy schedule, but it's worth it. The difference you will see and feel is well worth the time investment you make in the program.

I find that using the following suggestions makes my life a lot easier. I hope it will make your journey to health, or what I call UltraWellness, a little easier too.

PLAN YOUR MEALS AND SHOP IN ADVANCE

With the recipes in *The Blood Sugar Solution* and *The Blood Sugar Solution Cookbook,* you now have access to a great deal of variety in terms of what you eat while you are on the program. However, if you wait to decide what to eat until just before you leave for work or just after you get home in the evening, you are going to face a lot of temptation to cheat. The more you do that, the greater the danger of going off the program entirely.

My recommendation? Plan ahead of time. Take a few minutes one day per week to sit down and plan your meals for the upcoming week, and make a shopping list. Then go to the grocery store and purchase all of the ingredients for those recipes in advance.

You can do this and still leave enough flexibility to choose different meals on different days. Sit down on, say, a Sunday afternoon, and plan the next seven breakfasts, seven lunches, and seven dinners. Go shopping and buy your ingredients all at once. Then you can decide which of these meals you want to prepare and eat on any given day.

You can always run back to the store after work one evening if you decide you really want those grilled shrimp brochettes instead of the meal you had planned for that evening. But at least you will always have a healthy backup at home, waiting to be prepared.

PREPARE FOOD IN ADVANCE

When you come home tired from work, the last thing you want to do is spend a lot of time in the kitchen preparing food. But if you do part of the prep work and cooking in advance, it will reduce your time in the kitchen on any given evening, making it that much more likely that you'll prepare the meal you had planned rather than whipping up something quick that's less healthy, or getting take-out.

Here are a few tips on how to do this:

- **Cook on Sundays and Wednesdays.** Choose two days during the week (I find that Sunday and Wednesday work well for many people) when you are going to spend a few extra hours in the kitchen, cooking and preparing as much as you can in advance.
- **Prepare vegetables in advance.** You can cut and even steam your vegetables in advance, keep them in zipper-top bags, and then pull them out when you need them.
- **Clean and prepare meats in advance.** If you are cooking fish and shellfish, you can often do part of the prep work for these in advance as well. Devein your shrimp. Slice your fish into fillets that are the correct weight. Then freeze these items and pull them out when you need them.
- **Prepare sauces and marinades in advance.** If you're going to use a recipe that requires a sauce, vinaigrette, or marinade, you can always prepare these in advance, store them in glass containers in the

refrigerator, and pull them out during the week when you're ready to use them.

- **Cook brown rice and other whole grains in advance.** You can cook many whole grains, like brown rice, in advance. Keep them in your fridge and heat them up as needed.

BUY PREPARED PRODUCTS (BUT ONLY IF YOU HAVE TO)

While I usually recommend using fresh vegetables, beans, fish, and other products as much as possible, I am aware that when you are on a tight schedule, prepared products can be a lifesaver.

With the growing demand for high-quality prepared foods, you can now find many premium products that have been prepared in advance at stores like Whole Foods Market or Trader Joe's.

In the resources section on page 345, you will find a list of mail-order resources for high-quality organic fruits, vegetables, beans, grass-fed meats, and other excellent products. Here are a few specific ideas:

- **Use organic frozen vegetables** if you do not have time to prepare and cook vegetables. Choose organic, and choose a wide variety of different types of vegetables. Cascadian Farm provides high-quality organic frozen vegetables—almost as good as fresh.
- **Use canned beans, stocks, and other products such as sardines, artichokes, and roasted red peppers.** Make sure you stick to low-sodium versions of these as much as possible to keep the salt content of your diet down. Also, make sure to read the labels carefully to determine what ingredients are in the products you purchase.
- **Use canned wild Alaskan salmon** as your protein source at any meal. My favorite brand is Vital Choice (vitalchoice.com).
- **Stock up on jarred vegetables** such as artichokes, roasted red peppers, hearts of palm, and even sauerkraut (choose products in glass jars). These are quick and tasty ways to get extra vegetables into your diet.

Simple Cooking Tips

While most of the recipes in this cookbook are quick and easy to prepare, there are some very simple alternative cooking options you can take advantage of if you are absolutely stuck for time. Below are a few basic cooking techniques that will allow you to make quick meals according to the principles of the Blood Sugar Solution.

COOKING VEGETABLES

Steam or sauté your vegetables and add some fresh spices.

TO STEAM:

- Put 1 cup water in the bottom of a saucepan and bring it to a boil.
- Place a steaming rack or basket over the water (you can get one at any grocery store for about $2).
- Chop your veggies, place them in the steaming rack, cover, and steam them for 4–8 minutes, depending on the vegetable and your desired level of tenderness.
- Add your favorite seasonings, and drizzle with extra-virgin olive oil and a little sea salt to taste. You can cook almost any vegetable this way. It's easy. It's delicious. And it takes almost no time at all.

TO SAUTÉ:

- Put 1 tablespoon extra-virgin olive oil in the bottom of a frying pan. Turn the heat to medium high.
- Chop your veggies and drop them in.
- Sauté for 5–7 minutes, to your desired flavor and tenderness.

You can add onions, garlic, and/or mushrooms (shiitake are particularly tasty) to sautéed veggies to make them more flavorful. You might want to sauté your onions, garlic, and mushrooms first with a little salt, then drop in your chopped veggies.

COOKING FISH AND CHICKEN

Fish and chicken are very simple to prepare in a delicious and healthy way. Just grill, broil, or sauté your fish or boneless, skinless chicken, then season with olive oil, lemon juice, rosemary, garlic, ginger, or cilantro (I like to experiment with spices). Here's how:

TO BROIL OR GRILL:
- Preheat the broiler or grill.
- Sprinkle some sea salt and any other seasoning you choose on your fish or chicken. Place it under the broiler or on the grill.
- Cook fish until it is tender and opaque throughout, 7–10 minutes, flipping it once halfway through the cooking time. Chicken will take longer, perhaps up to 15 minutes. Again, flip it halfway. You will know it's done when you press the chicken with your finger and it's relatively firm, and it should be white throughout when you slice into it.

TO SAUTÉ:
- Sprinkle some sea salt and any other seasoning you choose on your fish or chicken.
- Put 1–2 tablespoons extra-virgin olive oil in the bottom of a frying pan. Turn the heat to medium-high to heat the oil. Place your fish or chicken in the pan.
- Turn fish just once while cooking, but turn chicken often to avoid browning it too much on one side. Follow the same cooking times as for broiling and grilling.

You could sauté onions, garlic, mushrooms, or even vegetables along with your fish or chicken to make it interesting.

Once it is cooked, season your fish or chicken with additional sea salt, up to 1 tablespoon extra-virgin olive oil, and lemon juice if you choose.

TOFU

Follow the same guidelines for fish and chicken, or simply add cubed tofu to your vegetables before steaming or sautéing.

BEANS

Rinse and drain your favorite canned beans (I prefer the small white cannellini or navy beans). Heat them in a saucepan with 1–2 tablespoons extra-virgin olive oil, rosemary, and sea salt. Add sautéed, chopped vegetables to the beans if you like. Be creative.

RICE

To cook brown or black rice, bring 4 cups filtered water to a boil. Rinse 2 cups uncooked brown or black rice, put it in the water with 1 tablespoon extra-virgin olive oil and ½ teaspoon sea salt, and cover. Bring to a boil and then simmer on the lowest heat, covered, for 45 minutes. Do not stir. Remember to limit your servings of grains to no more than ½ cup of cooked grain.

SPICE UP YOUR FOOD

Remember to add spices to your cooking. Place some slices of ginger in the water while you're cooking rice, or add 1–2 teaspoons turmeric for delicious yellow, Indian-style rice. These are powerful anti-inflammatories and give the rice a wonderful aroma and flavor. Add fresh rosemary, chopped fresh cilantro, or fresh crushed garlic to your vegetables.

Then serve. That's all there is to it.

You don't have to follow fancy recipes or spend hours in the kitchen every night to eat the Blood Sugar Solution way. Just stick to real, whole, allergen-free foods, and you'll watch the pounds come off as you approach UltraWellness.

How to Eat Out Safely

While I recommend that you avoid eating out on the Blood Sugar Solution program, I understand that this is sometimes impossible. Some people are obligated to go to business luncheons, for example. In that case, I recommend you follow these guidelines when eating out:

- Ask for grilled fish or chicken.
- Ask for a large plate of vegetables, either steamed with a side of sliced lemons and olive oil or sautéed in olive oil.

- You may have a salad, but skip the dressing and ask for extra-virgin olive oil and sliced lemons instead. Ask for some grilled chicken, shrimp, or salmon on top of your salad.

The Power of Mindful Eating

Take time to notice how every bite of your food looks, feels, and tastes in your mouth. When you think about what you are about to eat, how does it make you feel? What sensations does the aroma invoke? Savoring your meal is an act of gratitude toward your body and the earth. When we eat unconsciously we eat more. Avoid multitasking while eating. Turn off the phone, TV, email, and computer and take a break from media while you focus on nourishing yourself.

Follow these steps to practice mindful eating:

- **"Take Five" before a meal.** In one minute transform your metabolism by taking five slow breaths. Breathe in through your nose and count to five; pause; breathe out through your mouth and count to five. Repeat four more times or until you feel relaxed and ready to begin your meal.
- **Offer gratitude** before your meal.
- **Bring your attention** fully to the food.
- **Follow the 20-Minute Rule.** It takes 20 minutes for your stomach to tell your brain that it is full. If you eat quickly, you can easily overeat. So take your time. Put your fork down between bites. Chew your food well. Your digestion and metabolism—and your waistline—will thank you.

I encourage you to read two extraordinary books about the psychology of eating that can help you address the emotional and psychological barriers to true self-care and eating well. They are both by Marc David: *Nourishing Wisdom* and *The Slow Down Diet.*

3

Eat Your Medicine: Principles of Eating Healthy for Life

UNJUNK YOUR LIFE

Do not underestimate the power of removing addictive substances from your body. In order to do this effectively, you will need to clean out your pantry of all the junk. Benjamin Franklin said that "an ounce of prevention is worth a pound of cure." That has never been truer than for those with diabesity. By the time you have late-stage or even early diabesity, you need a pound of cure. If you have advanced diabesity, you need 10 pounds of cure!

This program is designed to reset and reboot your biology and metabolism. That is why you have to unjunk your diet, which will unjunk your metabolism. Eventually you may be able to enjoy a wider range of food and treats. Your body is the best barometer. If you get cravings or gain weight (or aren't losing weight), it's time to reassess how foods that raise your blood sugar may be sneaking in. Is it too much sweet potato, or that little bit of honey, or worse? Get focused and get healthy again.

UNJUNK YOUR DIET

Cut out:

- **Sugars in all forms,** from syrups, nectars, and honey to Stevia, sucralose, and xylitol. If you have to ask, "Is this okay?" *it isn't.* Small amounts (¼ to ½ cup) of alcohol in cooking are fine.

- **Flours in all forms,** including seemingly benign gluten-free flour. Avoid bagels, wraps, pasta, pastries, bread, etc.
- **All processed food.** Stay away from toxic factory-made "foodlike substances." Most packaged food consists of sugar, corn, flour, and soybean oil combined with chemicals, all shaped into different sizes and colors. It is injection-molded food, not fit for human consumption.
- **Gluten and dairy.** Avoid all forms, and remember to read ingredient labels for hidden sources.

If you are on the Advanced Plan: Avoid all grains, starchy vegetables (beets, sweet potatoes, parsnips, potatoes, rutabagas, taro, turnips, winter squash, etc.), and all fruit (except ½ cup of berries per day).

CREATE THE PERFECT PLATE

There is one key principle to remember as you use the recipes in this book and put together your meals every day. You want to create the perfect plate. This will balance your blood sugar by allowing you to feel full from eating an unlimited amount of low-glycemic vegetables along with a moderate amount of protein (the size of the palm of your hand), a small amount of whole-grain or starchy vegetables, and a small amount (½ cup) of fruit as a treat. If there is a dish containing grains, sweet potatoes, or squash, the serving size should be only ½ cup and fill only ¼ of your plate.

Here's how to create the perfect plate:

- 50 percent low-starch, low-glycemic vegetables (see list on page 33)
- 25 percent lean and clean protein (fish, chicken, eggs, meat, beans, nuts, seeds, and whole soy)
- 25 percent slow-burning carbohydrates (gluten-free whole grains, sweet potatoes, and winter squash)

If you are on the Advanced Plan, make your plate 75 percent low-starch vegetables and 25 percent protein; skip the grains and starchy veggies.

EAT ON TIME

Timing is everything when it comes to your metabolism. Not eating breakfast or eating too late can wreak havoc on your hormones and cause you to store fat instead of lose it. Pay attention to when you eat. Get into a regular rhythm. Your body loves consistency.

- **Avoid eating like a sumo wrestler.** Sumo wrestlers gain weight by eating a big meal right before bed. You should always have a protein-based breakfast within one hour of waking up, eat a protein-based lunch and dinner, and have a small protein-based snack, such as nuts or seeds, midmorning and midafternoon. Stop eating at least three hours before retiring to bed.
- **Establish your rhythm and stick to it.** Your body evolved and exists today because of natural rhythms. Stick to a rhythm and a schedule of when you wake up, when you go to bed, when you exercise, and especially when you eat; this will optimize digestion, power up your metabolism, and synchronize your hormones.

EAT YOUR MEDICINE

Choose SLOW Carbs, Not LOW Carbs

Fiber added to any meal reduces the glycemic load and prevents spikes in blood sugar and insulin. Aim for 30–50 grams daily. As with a stoplight, let green, yellow, or red be your guide.

GREEN CARBS: EAT FREELY

- **Fill half your plate with slow-burning, low-GL vegetables** such as arugula, asparagus, bell peppers, bok choy, broccoli, Brussels sprouts, cauliflower, celery, cucumbers, dandelion greens, hearts of palm, kale, lettuce, mushrooms, radishes, snap peas, tomatoes, watercress, etc.

- **Seaweed.** Kombu, nori, and wakame are all extraordinarily high in minerals, protein, and healing compounds. For more information on seaweed, create an account at drhyman.com/register, then go to the "Eat Your Medicine: Nutrition Basics for Everyone" report in the Downloads section.
- **Try shirataki noodles.** Made from konjac root (don't buy the ones made from tofu), they have lots of sugar-busting fiber and no carbs or calories. Yes, that's right—noodles with no calories!

YELLOW CARBS: EAT IN MODERATION

- **Whole grains.** Amaranth, brown and black rice, buckwheat, millet, quinoa, teff. Avoid all grains if you are on the Advanced Plan.
- **Legumes.** Adzuki beans, black beans, black-eyed peas, butter beans/baby lima beans, cannellini beans, chickpeas/garbanzo beans, fava beans/broad beans, Great Northern beans, kidney beans, lentils, mung beans, navy beans, pinto beans, split peas. Limit to ⅓ cup per serving if you are on the Advanced Plan. Avoid legumes if you are not making progress on the program, if you are extremely insulin resistant, or if you have digestive issues.
- **Dark berries.** Blackberries, raspberries, strawberries, wild blueberries. Limit to ½ cup daily if you are on the Advanced Plan.
- **Stone fruit.** Apricots, nectarines, peaches, plums. Avoid these if you are on the Advanced Plan.
- **Apples and pears.** Avoid these if you are on the Advanced Plan.

RED CARBS: EAT LIMITED AMOUNTS

- **Starchy, high-glycemic cooked vegetables.** Parsnips, pumpkins, sweet potatoes/yams, winter squash.
- **High-sugar fruits.** Bananas, grapes, melons, pineapple. Avoid all fruit juice or fruit packed in juice.

FORBIDDEN CARBS: AVOID COMPLETELY

- **Processed carbs.** Flour-based foods such as bagels, bread, cakes, cookies, crackers, muffins, and pizza. You have to be careful, because even healthy-sounding words like "whole-wheat" or "gluten-free" don't always equal authentic health foods. Foods such as whole-wheat bread or gluten-free pasta can wreak just as much havoc on blood sugar as their "white" counterparts—or even more. You know food is healthy when you can picture it growing in its natural state. Ask yourself how many steps were involved in creating the food. For example, compare an apple and apple juice. You can picture an apple growing in nature, and it has had nothing done to it before reaching your shopping cart, while the apple juice has been processed, treated, heated, flavored, etc.—you get the idea.
- **Gluten-containing whole grains.** Barley, einkorn, kamut, oats, rye, spelt, triticale, wheat.
- **Dried fruit.** Cranberries, dates, raisins, etc.

Boost Phytonutrient Intake: Choose Dark-Colored Plant Foods

Real food and spices are full of health-promoting phytonutrients. These molecules don't just taste good, they literally boost your metabolism and upgrade your biological software. Use them liberally! Here are the compounds, and their sources, that make food medicine:

allicin—garlic, onions
anthocyanidins—berries, black rice
beta-sitosterols—avocados, brown rice
capsaicin—chile peppers
catechins—tea (white tea is highest in antioxidants; green tea is a great option, too)
cinnamic acid—aloe, cinnamon
curcumin—turmeric
DIM (diindolylmethane)—broccoli family
ellagic acid—berries, walnuts
gingerol—ginger

glucosinolates—broccoli family
isoflavones—soy
kaempferol—broccoli, strawberries
lignans—broccoli, flaxseeds, sesame seeds
omega-3, -6, and -9 fatty acids—borage oil, sea vegetables
phytosterols—nuts, seeds
prebiotic—inulin from Jerusalem artichokes
probiotic— kimchi, sauerkraut
quercetin—apples, onions
resveratrol—grape skins
rutin—lemons, parsley
salicylic acid—peppermint
saponins—beans, quinoa
silymarin—artichokes, milk thistle
sulfides—garlic, onions, shallots
tocopherols—vitamin E from whole grains

Fat Does Not Make You Fat

Get an oil change. Replace bad fat with good fat.

While carbs are not "essential," fats are. Without enough of the right type of fats, your biology breaks down. Fats make up your cell walls. If you don't get enough or if you eat too much of the wrong kind, you will not have the building blocks required for healthy cell membranes, which you need for optimal insulin function and blood sugar control. Omega-3s are the king among healthy fats. In fact, 60 percent of your brain should be made from healthy omega-3 fats.

It can take a year to rebuild and remake all your cells and tissues with the right fats, so start right away. Choose anti-inflammatory fats such as omega-3 and monounsaturated fats over refined vegetable oils, trans fats, and hydrogenated fats.

- **Omega-3 fats.** Wild or sustainably raised cold-water fish such as salmon, sardines, herring, and other low-mercury fish. See nrdc.org for a list of the fish lowest in mercury.

- **Monounsaturated fats.** Olives, olive oil, avocados, almonds.
- **Healthy oil choices.** Extra-virgin olive oil; walnut and flaxseed oil for salads; sesame, grapeseed, and sunflower oil for baking.
- **Healthy saturated fat.** Enjoy plant-based extra-virgin coconut butter in place of butter. It is full of medium-chain triglycerides, the perfect fuel for your cells and your brain, and contains anti-inflammatory, immune-boosting lauric acid (also found in breast milk).

Eat High-Quality Protein: The Key to Controlling Hunger and Losing Weight

Many studies, such as those outlined in T. Colin Campbell's book *The China Study*, point to the risks of too much animal protein. However, these studies are based mostly on factory-produced animal protein, not the wild species that made up the diet of our hunter-gatherer ancestors. The wild elk and deer meat my patients gave me when I was a small-town doctor in Idaho had very different nutritional properties and fats from those of a feedlot cow.

Some people thrive as vegans, others wither. Some feel great when eating animal protein, others get sick and sluggish. You need to find out what works for your body, and this will take some experimentation. My experience with patients with diabesity is that they typically need more good-quality animal protein (grass- or range-fed animals, free-range eggs, or sustainably farmed or wild low-mercury fish).

Whether you choose vegetarian or animal sources, it is essential that you get protein at each meal and snack. It turns up your metabolic fire and ability to burn calories while reducing your appetite. Try:

- Beans or legumes (but be aware that they can spike blood sugar and insulin in some).
- Whole soy products such as tofu or tempeh. Choose non-GMO and organic; avoid industrially processed soy, including soy burgers, hot dogs, and sausage.
- Nuts and seeds.
- Omega-3 or free-range eggs.

- Mercury-free fish, shrimp, and scallops.
- Organic, grass-fed, and hormone-, antibiotic-, and pesticide-free poultry.
- Wild game and lean, clean red meat in small portions. See ewg.org/meateatersguide for ways to safely eat meat and reduce both the adverse health effects on your health as well as the impact on the environment and the planet.

Use Herbs, Spices, and Other Seasonings to Add Flavor and Make Your Meals Come Alive

- Wheat-free tamari, red chile paste (Sriracha is great, but get a brand without sulfites and preservatives), tahini, exotic spices, sea salt, peppercorns, fresh herbs, and homemade or store-bought organic, gluten-free, low-sodium broth or stock.
- Canned or jarred foods: salmon, sardines, tomatoes, beans, artichokes, and red peppers.

BEWARE OF HIDDEN FOOD ALLERGIES AND SENSITIVITIES

Food is information for your body, and some foods have the wrong information for some people, so take note of which foods affect you negatively. Gluten and dairy are the most common suspects. They are inflammatory; for some the inflammation causes weight gain and diabesity. Read *The Blood Sugar Solution* for an in-depth exploration into the many health problems that these two common food allergens may pose for you. Avoid gluten and dairy for six weeks, and you might not only lose weight, but many other nagging chronic symptoms and pains may just go away. It is a profound and powerful experiment, and I encourage you to try it and let your body tell you what it needs.

SAFELY REINTRODUCE GLUTEN AND DAIRY

All of the recipes in this book are safe for you to eat except for those in Chapter 6, which reintroduce gluten and dairy. After Week 6 you will want to challenge your system with certain foods to see how your body responds. The two foods you need to consider reintegrating are gluten and dairy. Here's how to properly reintroduce them into your diet without sabotaging success:

OPTION 1: STAY OFF GLUTEN AND DAIRY COMPLETELY

You might feel better on this program than you've ever felt in your life. If this is true for you, chances are you have some level of sensitivity to these commonly allergenic foods. Despite what you have been told by the food industry, your body actually can live just fine without gluten and dairy. *If it feels right to go without, listen to that inner wisdom and stay off them!* After you have reset your metabolism and found what foods and lifestyle choices nourish you, treats or small tastes of these foods should be all right, assuming you do not have a life-threatening reaction to them or they don't trigger compulsive overeating for you.

OPTION 2: REINTRODUCE GLUTEN AND DAIRY

Are you curious about how gluten and dairy affect your body? I hope so! I encourage you to investigate how these foods make you feel and influence your health. Your own body is the best indicator of what it likes and what it doesn't, what makes it feel good or feel bad. You need to listen to your body and pay attention to how it reacts to gluten and dairy. This information helps you understand what contributes to your health and what diminishes it. There is a way to slowly and safely reintroduce these foods without reversing all the progress you have made. This is my system:

1. Start with dairy.
2. Eat it at least 2–3 times a day for 3 days.
3. Track your reactions for those 3 days.
4. If you have a reaction, stop dairy immediately.
5. Wait 3 days.
6. Now try gluten. Repeat steps 2–5 and remember to quit if you experience a reaction.

You might experience the following when you add these foods back into your diet:

- weight gain
- cravings
- fluid retention
- nasal congestion
- chest congestion
- headaches
- brain fog
- difficulty remembering things
- mood problems
- sleep problems
- joint aches
- muscle aches
- pain
- fatigue
- changes in your skin (acne, eczema)
- changes in digestion or bowel function (bloating, gas, diarrhea, constipation, or reflux)

Some people react immediately and others have a delayed reaction. If you don't experience a reaction within 72 hours, you should be safe. If you do experience a reaction, then I suggest you eliminate the food from your diet for 3 months. Some of you may need to eliminate it for 6 months and work with a qualified dietitian or nutritionally oriented physician to help cool the inflammation and heal your gut.

You can use the food log opposite to track reactions to any foods you eat. In the column on the left, note the date you ate the food. In the middle column, describe the food itself. And in the column on the right, describe the symptoms you experienced (use the preceding list as a guide to what to look for). If you do this consistently, you will soon develop a picture of which foods are causing you health problems and weight gain.

Food Allergy Reintroduction Log		
DATE	**FOOD INTRODUCED**	**SYMPTOMS**

Trust Your Body's Nutritional Wisdom

Moderation, variety, and balance are paramount to lifelong health. Wellness is about knowing what serves you. There will always be some new diet fad or trend in health, yet the ability to understand what nourishes your unique system is the result of self-awareness and self-care.

Regardless of your level of tolerance to common food allergens like gluten and dairy, focus on taking small portions of these foods just a couple of times of week so that you don't have to revisit the vicious cycle of food allergies and inflammation. And when you eat, do so with attention to your whole body so that you are present to its signals and feedback. Be open to tuning in and hearing your body's message.

Avoid Food Emergencies

When you are hungry, there are a load of "junk food" alternatives in convenience stores and fast-food restaurants. Stay away from them! I encourage you to create an emergency life pack of food. Watch this video as I share with you what I have in my Emergency Life Pack: drhyman.com/blog/video/dr-hymans-emergency-food-pack/.

A WORD ON THE RECIPES

The recipes in the following chapters come from my own kitchen and from the kitchens of my family, friends, and the online UltraWellness community. Each recipe has been approved by me. Some recipes, especially those in the reintroduction phase, have a little more starch or sugar, which is fine. Once you have rebooted your metabolism you can tolerate an occasional treat.

The Difference between the Basic, Advanced, and Reintroduction Recipes

The Basic Plan recipes (Chapter 4) are designed to be used by everyone and will prevent and reverse early diabesity. If the whole country ate this way, most chronic disease would be eliminated. The Advanced Plan recipes (Chapter 5) are designed for those with advanced diabesity (based on the quiz) and those with type 2 diabetes. These recipes are based on whole foods, vegetables, lean protein, nuts and seeds, and small amounts of fruit. The Advanced Plan eliminates all sugar and insulin-spiking high-glycemic foods including, of course, sugar in any form, grains, starchy vegetables, and all but ½ cup of berries a day. After you have reversed advanced diabesity and your weight and numbers are normal, you may be able to switch to the Basic Plan.

While I think most of us would be better off eating very little (or no) dairy or gluten, some may tolerate these foods in moderation. That is why Chapter 6 includes reintroduction recipes, which introduce gluten and dairy back into your diet. Careful reintroduction of dairy and gluten is essential to identify any hidden food sensitivities. Desserts are included as occasional treats (Chapter 7), but they are not intended to be eaten daily or in anything other than small amounts. Watch your reaction, watch your body. Notice how you respond. If these treats trigger a cycle of sugar cravings and bingeing, it is better to stay away. Eventually, as you reboot your metabolism, you should have the ability to enjoy them from time to time.

How Cost Was Estimated

As I've mentioned before, eating well can fit into any budget. We all deserve to eat a clean diet, and I hope you heed the advice I gave earlier about how to accomplish this.

How did I estimate cost per recipe in this cookbook? Quite simply, I looked at the total yield of a recipe and divided it by how many servings it provides. Each recipe budget is based on what one serving would cost. I gave special attention to those recipes that were able to yield several servings and feed a large group or feed you for several meals. So even if an ingredient is somewhat pricey, if it is high quality and it lends itself to other meals or stretches out through many servings, then overall, it is cost efficient and warrants a low-budget estimate.

While I took the cost and value of each recipe into careful consideration, most important is for you to make these delicious meals work for you and your needs. If you find an ingredient that makes even better sense for your budget, please don't be afraid to experiment and see what you come up with. Creating recipes is an art—have fun, keep an open mind, and allow creativity to help you overcome any barriers to success.

How Level of Ease Was Estimated

I understand that some of you might be novices in the kitchen and this may be your first time really picking up a recipe to follow in earnest. To that end, I want to ensure that your journey through *The Blood Sugar Solution Cookbook* is a safe and exciting learning experience. I modified certain recipes to ensure that you would find the recipes easy to prepare and well organized, regardless of your talent or culinary expertise. You will see that only a small handful of the recipes are designated as moderately difficult to prepare. I hope this allows you to sit back, relax, and enjoy the ride. Be creative, garner patience, and take it slowly. What seemed challenging yesterday might seem effortless tomorrow!

PART II

THE RECIPES

4

The Basic Plan

INTRODUCTION

The Basic Plan is designed for those with mild diabesity, those who are just beginning down the road to pre-diabetes and diabetes. Taking the quiz on page 10 will help you select the best starting place for doing the Blood Sugar Solution and guide you toward the best use of this cookbook.

The Basic Plan includes small amounts (½ cup a day) of gluten-free whole grains such as brown or black rice, quinoa or buckwheat. It also allows for starchy vegetables such as sweet potatoes or winter squash and a little more variety of fruit. This is a plan that, in fact, can be followed for life by most people with an occasional treat (which is why I added the reintroduction and dessert sections!). Controlling insulin and blood sugar is the key to staying at a healthy weight and avoiding most of the disease of aging, including heart disease, stroke, dementia, and even many cancers. Your body will be the best guide and indicator of success. It is the best feedback system for what works and what doesn't.

If you find you follow the Basic Plan, and don't get the results you want in terms of health, weight loss, or blood sugar control, then move to the Advanced Plan. Of course, you can combine recipes from any section and may use any recipes in the Advanced section if you are on the Basic Plan, and I encourage you to do so for variety and fun.

BREAKFAST

ULTRASHAKE

Serves: 1

Prep time:
5 minutes

Level: Easy

Budget: $

This shake provides all of the essential protein, omega-3 fatty acids, fiber, antioxidants, and phytonutrients for detoxification. It will balance your blood sugar and help you maintain a healthy blood sugar level throughout the day.

- 2 scoops rice, hemp, or pea protein powder (any good quality plant protein powder will do)
- 1 tablespoon flaxseed oil–borage oil combination
- 2 tablespoons ground flaxseeds
- ½ cup frozen or fresh noncitrus fruit such as blueberries, cherries, raspberries, peaches, pears, or strawberries
- 6 ounces water
- 1 tablespoon nut butter (almond, macadamia, cashew, pecan, or sunflower seed) or ¼ cup nuts (such as almonds, walnuts, pecans, cashews, or any combination) soaked in water overnight (optional)
- handful of ice if using non-frozen fruit

Combine all of the ingredients in a blender. Blend on high speed until smooth, about 2 minutes. If the shake is too thick, add more water until you reach a thick but drinkable consistency.

Nutritional analysis per serving (1 cup): calories 377, fat 17 g, saturated fat 3 g, cholesterol 0 mg, fiber 14 g, protein 12 g, carbohydrate 47 g, sodium 129 mg

POPEYE THE SAILOR ENERGY BOOST

This is a wonderful breakfast, full of unusual breakfast ingredients, including chia seeds, avocados, and spinach mixed up into a super smoothie with the right amount of phytochemicals and protein. And it's low in sugar, too.

- 1 cup water
- 1 cup unsweetened almond milk
- 1 small apple, cored
- flesh of ½ avocado
- ½ tablespoon chia seeds
- 1 date, pitted
- juice of ½ lemon
- 2 cups baby spinach
- ½ teaspoon ground cinnamon
- 4 ice cubes

Serves: 2

Prep time: 5 minutes

Level: Easy

Budget: $

Combine all of the ingredients in a blender and blend on high speed until smooth, 1–2 minutes. If the shake is too thick, thin it with more ice or almond milk—it should be thick but drinkable. Serve chilled.

Nutritional analysis per serving (1 cup): calories 166, fat 10 g, saturated fat 1 g, cholesterol 0 mg, fiber 8 g, protein 3 g, carbohydrate 24 g, sodium 118 mg

Raspberry Banana Cream Pie Smoothie

Serves: 2

Prep time:
5 minutes

Level: Easy

Budget: $

A creative way to eat your greens along with phytochemicals from berries.

- ½ cup frozen blueberries
- ⅓ cup frozen raspberries
- 4 frozen strawberries
- ½ large frozen banana
- 10 unsalted almonds
- 8 walnuts
- ½ teaspoon spirulina powder
- 1 teaspoon green powder

Combine all of the ingredients in a blender and add just enough water to cover them. Blend on high speed until smooth, 1–2 minutes. If the smoothie is too thick, thin it with a little water—it should be thick but drinkable. Serve chilled.

Nutritional analysis per serving (½ cup): calories 178, fat 8 g, saturated fat 1 g, cholesterol 0 mg, fiber 6 g, protein 6 g, carbohydrate 25 g, sodium 22 mg

Green Chia Porridge

Combining nuts, avocados, chia seeds, spinach, and berries in a blender makes a fantastic and satisfying breakfast.

- 1 cup water
- 5 almonds (soaked), walnuts, or cashews
- flesh of ½ avocado
- ½ banana
- 1 tablespoon chia seeds
- 1½ cups baby spinach
- ¼ cup raspberries, for garnish
- 1 tablespoon bee pollen (optional, for garnish)

Serves: 1

Prep time: 5 minutes

Level: Easy

Budget: $

Combine the water, nuts, avocado, banana, chia seeds, and spinach in a blender. Blend on high speed until smooth and creamy. Garnish with raspberries and bee pollen (if using) and serve.

Nutritional analysis per serving (2 cups): calories 316, fat 18 g, saturated fat 2 g, cholesterol 0 mg, fiber 14 g, protein 10 g, carbohydrate 40 g, sodium 53 mg

DR. HYMAN'S CHINESE EGGS AND GREENS

Serves: 3
Prep time: 15 minutes
Cook time: 20 minutes
Level: Easy
Budget: $

A savory way to enjoy omega-3 eggs. The juiciness of the tomatoes makes this feel like an indulgent breakfast, but it takes only minutes to prepare. Cooking tomatoes in a little healthy oil enhances their nutritional value and increases the availability of their potent cancer-fighting lycopene.

- 3 tablespoons extra-virgin olive oil
- 12 garlic cloves, chopped
- 6 large eggs, beaten
- 1 (16-ounce) can chopped plum tomatoes, undrained
- 1 tablespoon toasted sesame oil
- 1 tablespoon reduced-sodium, gluten-free tamari
- 1 teaspoon Worcestershire sauce
- 1 cup cooked black rice
- 6 cups baby spinach, pre-steamed

1. Heat the oil in a large nonstick pan or wok over medium-high heat. Add the garlic and cook until aromatic, 1–2 minutes.

2. Pour the eggs into the pan and cook them, undisturbed, until no egg liquid remains. This takes about 1–2 minutes. Flip the omelet over carefully and cook the other side for 1–2 minutes. When cooked through, use a spatula to cut the omelet into 2-inch pieces.

3. Pour the tomatoes, along with their juices, over the eggs and add the sesame oil, tamari, and Worcestershire sauce. Simmer the eggs in the sauce for 10 minutes.

4. Remove the pan from the heat and serve the eggs and tomatoes over black rice with steamed spinach on the side. Leftover eggs can be refrigerated for up to 2 days.

Nutritional analysis per serving (¾ cup egg mixture, ⅓ cup rice): calories 462, fat 29 g, saturated fat 6 g, cholesterol 430 mg, fiber 4 g, protein 20 g, carbohydrate 36 g, sodium 532 mg

SOUPS

HEARTY LENTIL SOUP

Serves: 4

Prep time:
10 minutes

Cook time:
35 minutes

Level: Easy

Budget: $

Lentils are a wonderful source of minerals, nutrients, fiber, and protein, and they are a staple in many cultures. They provide a nutty, sweet, deeply satisfying flavor.

- 1 tablespoon extra-virgin olive oil
- 1 teaspoon dried basil
- 1 small yellow onion, finely chopped
- 2 large carrots, peeled and finely chopped
- sea salt and freshly ground black pepper
- 8 cups low-sodium vegetable broth
- 1 cup dried lentils
- ⅓ cup uncooked long-grain brown rice
- 1 (28-ounce) can crushed tomatoes

1. Heat the oil in a medium pot over medium-high heat. After a minute add the basil and let it infuse for 30 seconds while stirring.

2. Add the onions and carrots and season to taste with salt and black pepper. Cook, stirring occasionally, until the vegetables are soft, 5–6 minutes.

3. Pour in the broth and add the lentils, rice, and tomatoes. Bring to a boil and reduce the heat to low. Simmer with the lid slightly ajar for 20–25 minutes.

4. Remove the pot from the heat and taste for seasoning. Add more salt and black pepper if desired. Serve immediately. Store any leftovers in the refrigerator for up to 4 days or in the freezer for up to 4 months.

Nutritional analysis per serving (1½ cups): calories 221, fat 3 g, saturated fat 0 g, cholesterol 0 mg, fiber 13 g, protein 11 g, carbohydrate 38 g, sodium 605 mg

HEARTY KALE STEW

Serves: 6

Prep time:
15 minutes

Cook time:
25 minutes

Level: Moderate

Budget: $

The rosemary, thyme, garlic, and turmeric in this comforting vegetable stew combine to help calm inflammation.

- 2 cups cooked red kidney beans or 1 (15-ounce) can red kidney beans, rinsed and drained
- 3 cups low-sodium chicken broth
- 1 cup dried lentils
- 1 large bunch kale, stemmed and chopped
- 1 (28-ounce) can diced tomatoes, undrained
- 4 celery ribs, chopped
- 2 medium yellow onions, chopped
- 4 large carrots, peeled and chopped
- 3 garlic cloves, minced
- 8 large portobello mushrooms, chopped
- 1 bay leaf
- 1 tablespoon dried rosemary
- 1 tablespoon dried thyme
- 1 tablespoon ground turmeric
- sea salt and freshly ground black pepper

1. Combine all of the ingredients in a medium pot, cover, and simmer gently until the lentils are cooked and the vegetables are very tender, 20–25 minutes.

2. Transfer half of the stew to a blender and blend on high speed until smooth, about 2 minutes. Pour the blended soup back into the pot with the remaining stew and stir until evenly combined. (Or use a handheld immersion blender to purée some of the soup right in the pot.) Check for seasoning and add salt and black pepper if desired. Serve hot. Any leftovers can be refrigerated for up to 4 days.

Nutritional analysis per serving (1 cup): calories 241, fat 1 g, saturated fat 0 g, cholesterol 0 mg, fiber 16 g, protein 14 g, carbohydrate 44 g, sodium 115 mg

BEAN SOUP

Serves: 8

Prep time:
20 minutes

Cook time:
45 minutes

Level: Easy

Budget: $

Bean soups are fabulous! They include good-quality plant protein, fiber, and minerals, and make a hearty, satisfying, easy-to-make meal that can be kept for days in the refrigerator.

- 2 cups cooked chickpeas or 1 (15-ounce) can chickpeas, rinsed and drained
- 2 cups cooked black beans or 1 (15-ounce) can black beans, rinsed and rained
- 1 cup dried lentils
- 8 cups low-sodium vegetable broth
- 3 tablespoons extra-virgin olive oil
- 1 large onion, chopped
- 6 garlic cloves, finely chopped
- 1 large tomato, chopped
- 1 medium carrot, peeled and chopped
- 3 celery ribs, chopped
- 12 shiitake mushrooms, stemmed and thinly sliced
- 3 scallions, thinly sliced
- 1 small bunch kale, stemmed and chopped
- 3 sprigs fresh thyme
- 1 teaspoon chili powder
- 1 teaspoon ground coriander
- ½ teaspoon ground cumin
- sea salt and freshly ground black pepper

1. Combine the chickpeas, black beans, lentils, and broth in a large soup pot and bring to a boil over high heat. Reduce the heat to low and simmer the soup, uncovered, for 15 minutes.

2. Meanwhile, heat the oil in a medium cast-iron pan over medium-high heat. Add the onions and cook until soft and brown, 5–7 minutes. Add the garlic and cook until aromatic, 1–2 minutes. Stir in the tomato and cook until soft, 6–8 minutes.

3. Stir in the carrot, celery, mushrooms, scallions, kale, thyme, chili powder, coriander, and cumin. Season the vegetables to taste with salt

and black pepper and cover the pan. Cook until the kale wilts and is tender, 6–8 minutes.

4. Stir the vegetables into the pot with the cooked beans and serve hot. Any leftovers can be stored in the refrigerator for up to 4 days or in the freezer for up to 6 months.

Nutritional analysis per serving (1 cup): calories 270, fat 6 g, saturated fat 1 g, cholesterol 0 mg, fiber 14 g, protein 14 g, carbohydrate 41 g, sodium 258 mg

ROASTED RED PEPPER AND CANNELLINI BEAN SOUP

This comforting, creamy soup is easy to prepare, kid-friendly, and great to have for leftovers. It is a plant-based protein, low in sugar, and gluten- and dairy-free, and it can be combined with a salad for a complete meal.

Serves: 12

Prep time: 15 minutes

Cook time: 15 minutes

Level: Easy

Budget: $

- 10 cups cooked cannellini beans or 6 (15-ounce) cans cannellini beans, rinsed and drained
- 6 cups low-sodium vegetable broth
- 3 large red bell peppers
- 3 tablespoons extra-virgin olive oil
- ½ bunch or 1½ ounces fresh basil, thinly sliced, plus whole basil leaves for garnish
- 3 garlic cloves, minced
- sea salt and freshly ground black pepper

1. Combine the beans and broth in a large pot and bring to a boil over high heat. Reduce the heat to low and simmer the beans for 10 minutes while you roast the peppers. (To save time, you can use jarred roasted red peppers.)

2. Coat the peppers with a little bit of the oil and set them over an open high flame. Turn them occasionally using a long pair of tongs. Once blackened all over, transfer the peppers to a large bowl and cover the bowl tightly with plastic wrap. Allow the peppers to cool in the bowl; the steam created by the hot peppers will moisten the skin and make peeling it much easier. When cool, peel and remove any charred skin. Cut the peppers in half and discard the seeds and stem.

3. Add the roasted peppers, basil, remaining oil, and garlic to the beans. Transfer the soup in batches to a blender and blend on high speed until smooth, about 2 minutes. (Or use a handheld immersion blender to purée the soup right in the pot.) Turn the heat to low to warm the soup and season it to taste with salt and black pepper. Serve garnished

with a basil leaf. Leftover soup can be refrigerated for up to 4 days or frozen for up to 4 months.

Nutritional analysis per serving (1 cup): calories 205, fat 5 g, saturated fat 1 g, cholesterol 0 mg, fiber 9 g, protein 11 g, carbohydrate 30 g, sodium 255 mg

BLISSFUL BUTTERNUT BISQUE

This creamy, flavorful vegan soup is full of vitamin B, fiber, and nutrients. It provides that sweet taste that we all love. Be sure to combine it with protein for a complete meal. Ghee is clarified butter used in South Asian cooking. Find it in Asian markets or natural foods stores.

- 1 tablespoon ghee
- 1 medium Vidalia onion, chopped
- ½ teaspoon dried sage
- 4 fresh sage leaves, chopped
- 1 large butternut squash, peeled, seeded, and chopped
- 6 cups low-sodium vegetable broth
- sea salt and freshly ground black pepper
- ½ cup unsweetened coconut milk
- 2 tablespoons toasted pumpkin seeds

Serves: 6

Prep time: 5 minutes

Cook time: 35 minutes

Level: Easy

Budget: $

1. Heat the ghee in a large pot over medium-high heat. After a minute, add the onion and sauté until translucent, 3–5 minutes.

2. Add the dried sage, fresh sage, and squash and cook until the squash begins to soften slightly, 4–5 minutes.

3. Pour in the broth and season the soup to taste with salt and black pepper.

4. Bring the soup to a boil, then reduce the heat to low and simmer until the squash is tender, about 20 minutes.

5. Transfer the soup in batches to a blender and blend on high speed until smooth, about 2 minutes. (Or use a handheld immersion blender to purée the soup right in the pot.) Put the pot over low heat to warm the soup, and stir in the coconut milk. Taste the soup for seasoning and add more salt and black pepper if desired.

6. Garnish each portion with a few toasted pumpkin seeds and serve immediately. Any leftovers can be stored in the refrigerator for up to 4 days or in the freezer for up to 4 months.

Nutritional analysis per serving (¾ cup): calories 107, fat 4 g, saturated fat 2 g, cholesterol 5 mg, fiber 4 g, protein 6 g, carbohydrate 15 g, sodium 114 mg

KAREN'S SOUTHWEST BLACK BEAN SOUP

Serves: 8

Prep time:
15 minutes

Cook time:
35 minutes

Level: Easy

Budget: $

This hearty, thick soup is accented with rich flavors from the chipotles and carried by the texture of the tomatoes. Make sure to finish with fresh parsley or cilantro and chopped red bell pepper to bring this soup to life.

- 3 tablespoons extra-virgin olive oil
- 3 tablespoons ground ancho chile powder
- 1 tablespoon dried oregano
- 2 teaspoons ground cumin
- 2 bay leaves
- 1 medium red onion, finely chopped
- 4 garlic cloves, minced
- 1 canned chipotle chile in adobo sauce (optional)
- 1 (15-ounce) can Italian whole peeled tomatoes
- 1 (15-ounce) can tomato sauce
- 1 (6-ounce) can tomato paste
- sea salt and freshly ground black pepper
- 6 cups low-sodium chicken broth
- 6 cups cooked black beans or 4 (15-ounce) cans black beans, rinsed and drained
- 1 large red bell pepper, seeded and finely chopped
- ¼ cup finely chopped fresh parsley or cilantro

1. Heat the oil in a large pot over medium heat. After a minute add the ancho chile powder, oregano, cumin, and bay leaves and toast them, stirring, for 30 seconds.

2. Add the onion, garlic, and chipotle pepper, if using, and cook, stirring frequently, until the onion is soft and coated in spices, 3–4 minutes.

3. Pour in the tomatoes, tomato sauce, and tomato paste and season to taste with salt and black pepper. Add the broth and black beans and turn up the heat to high. When the soup comes to a boil, immediately reduce it to a simmer.

4. Cook with the lid ajar for 25 minutes. Check for seasoning and add additional salt and black pepper if desired.

5. Serve each portion garnished with bell pepper and fresh parsley. Any leftovers can be stored in the refrigerator for up to 4 days or in the freezer for up to 4 months.

Nutritional analysis per serving (1½ cups): calories 282, fat 2 g, saturated fat 0 g, cholesterol 0 mg, fiber 12 g, protein 17 g, carbohydrate 51 g, sodium 536 mg

Slow Cooker Vegetarian Chili

Serves: 10

Prep time: 10 minutes

Cook time: 2 hours 10 minutes

Level: Easy

Budget: $

Chili is a wonderful way to combine spices, flavors, vegetables, and beans in a hearty, heartwarming, phytonutrient–rich meal. When a recipe calls for wine, it's fine to use because the alcohol will burn off during cooking while the flavor remains. If you prefer, you can replace red wine with a savory stock, such as chicken or beef, or red wine vinegar.

- 1 tablespoon extra-virgin olive oil
- 2 tablespoons chili powder
- 1 tablespoon dried oregano
- 1 tablespoon dried parsley
- 1 tablespoon dried basil
- 3 bay leaves
- 1 teaspoon paprika
- 1 teaspoon ground coriander
- 1 teaspoon ground cumin
- ¼ teaspoon cayenne pepper
- 1 small yellow onion, chopped
- 3 celery ribs, chopped
- 3 garlic cloves, minced
- ¾ cup cremini mushrooms, chopped
- 1 red bell pepper, seeded and chopped
- sea salt and freshly ground black pepper
- 2 cups cooked kidney beans or 1 (15-ounce) can kidney beans, rinsed and drained
- 2 cups cooked cannellini beans or 1 (15-ounce) can cannellini beans, rinsed and drained
- 2 cups cooked black beans or 1 (15-ounce) can black beans, rinsed and drained
- 2 (15-ounce) cans diced tomatoes, undrained
- 1 (15-ounce) can tomato sauce
- 1 cup uncooked quinoa
- ¼ cup medium-bodied red wine, such as Pinot Noir

- 1 cup low-sodium vegetable broth
- 1 avocado, peeled, pitted, and diced, for garnish
- ¼ cup fresh cilantro leaves, for garnish

1. In a large cast-iron pan, heat the oil over medium-high heat. After a minute add the herbs and spices and toast, stirring, for 30 seconds. Stir in the onion and celery and cook in the spice oil until soft, 5–6 minutes.

2. Add the garlic, mushrooms, and bell pepper. Season to taste with salt and black pepper and cook for 3–4 minutes.

3. Dump the sautéed vegetable mixture, along with the beans, tomatoes, tomato sauce, quinoa, wine, and broth into a slow cooker. Cover and cook on the Low setting for 2 hours. If you prefer to cook the chili on the stovetop, put a large Dutch oven over very low heat and cook with the lid slightly ajar for 1 hour.

4. Remove the bay leaves. Serve garnished with the diced avocado and cilantro leaves. Leftover chili can be stored in the refrigerator for up to 4 days or in the freezer for up to 4 months.

Nutritional analysis per serving (½ cup): calories 250, fat 3 g, saturated fat 0 g, cholesterol 0 mg, fiber 11 g, protein 11 g, carbohydrate 40 g, sodium 417 mg

VEGETABLE CHILI WITH SMOKED SPICES

Serves: 12

Prep time:
10 minutes

Cook time:
45 minutes

Level: Moderate

Budget: $$

Earthy and rich with diversity in texture and taste, this hearty vegetable chili is a great way to use low-glycemic vegetables in one simple and delicious dish.

- 2 tablespoons extra-virgin olive oil
- 2 tablespoons ground ancho chile powder
- 1 tablespoon smoked paprika
- 1 tablespoon ground cumin
- ½ teaspoon smoked black pepper
- ¼ teaspoon ground chipotle chile powder
- 1 tablespoon dried Italian herb blend (or any combination of dried oregano, thyme, rosemary, and basil)
- 1 medium onion, chopped
- 3 garlic cloves, minced
- 3 large carrots, peeled and chopped
- 1 large zucchini, seeded and chopped
- 1 medium yellow squash, chopped
- 3 (15-ounce) cans crushed tomatoes
- 2 cups cooked cannellini beans or 1 (15-ounce) can cannellini beans, rinsed and drained
- 2 cups cooked kidney beans or 1 (15-ounce) can kidney beans, rinsed and drained
- sea salt and freshly ground black pepper
- 1 bunch or 3 ounces fresh chives, finely chopped, for garnish

1. Heat the oil in a large pot over medium heat. Add the spices and toast, stirring, for 30 seconds.
2. Add the onion and garlic to the pot and cook in the spiced oil, stirring frequently, until the onion is softened, 5–6 minutes.
3. Toss in the carrots, zucchini, and yellow squash and cook, stirring, until soft, 6–7 minutes.
4. Pour in the tomatoes and beans and season to taste with salt and black pepper.

5. Cover the pot and reduce the heat so that the chili is gently simmering. Cook at a low simmer until all of the vegetables are tender, 25–30 minutes. Check for seasoning and add additional salt and black pepper if desired. Garnish each portion with a few chives and serve. Leftover chili can be refrigerated for up to 5 days or frozen for up to 4 months.

Nutritional analysis per serving (1 cup): calories 122, fat 3 g, saturated fat 0 g, cholesterol 0 mg, fiber 7 g, protein 6 g, carbohydrate 20 g, sodium 244 mg

SADIE'S WHITE BEAN AND SHRIMP SOUP

Serves: 10

Prep time:
10 minutes

Cook time:
35 minutes

Level: Moderate

Budget: $$

Tomato paste adds depth to this light and lean soup. The shrimp contribute a great source of lean protein to balance out the hearty beans. If you like it a little spicy, add a few shakes of red pepper flakes before serving.

- 2 tablespoons extra-virgin olive oil
- 1 large Vidalia onion, chopped
- 5 garlic cloves, minced
- ¼ cup tomato paste
- 2 tablespoons finely chopped fresh oregano
- red pepper flakes
- sea salt and freshly ground black pepper
- 6 cups low-sodium chicken broth
- 1 (28-ounce) can whole peeled tomatoes, undrained
- 4 cups cooked cannellini beans or 2 (15-ounce) cans cannellini beans, rinsed and drained
- ½ bunch or 1½ ounces fresh parsley, finely chopped
- 1 large bunch kale, stemmed and roughly chopped
- 1½ pounds raw shrimp, peeled and deveined
- 1 bunch or 2 ounces fresh basil, torn

1. Heat the oil in a large pot over medium-high heat. Add the onion and garlic and cook until soft, 3–4 minutes.

2. Stir in the tomato paste and cook until it browns to a rusty red color. Add the oregano and season to taste with red pepper flakes, salt, and black pepper.

3. Pour in ½ cup of the broth and lightly scrape the bottom of the pan with a wooden spoon to lift any browned bits of tomato paste. Cook until the liquid has reduced by half, 3–5 minutes.

4. Add the tomatoes, beans, and remaining 5½ cups broth and stir to combine. Bring the soup to a boil, reduce the heat to low, and simmer for 20–25 minutes.

5. Add the parsley, kale, and shrimp to the pot and season generously with salt and black pepper.

6. Cook until the shrimp are pink and firm, 2–3 minutes.

7. Remove from the heat and add half of the basil to the soup. Check for seasoning and add additional red pepper flakes, salt, or black pepper if desired.

8. Transfer the soup to a large serving bowl or ladle into individual bowls. Garnish with the basil and serve. Any leftovers can be refrigerated for up to 2 days or frozen for up to 2 months.

Nutritional analysis per serving (2 cups): calories 320, fat 7 g, saturated fat 1 g, cholesterol 147 mg, fiber 12 g, protein 27 g, carbohydrate 38 g, sodium 328 mg

HEALING CHICKEN SOUP

Serves: 4

Prep time: 5 minutes

Cook time: 45 minutes

Level: Easy

Budget: $

Soup allows you to combine different ingredients into a healing potion. The ginger, curry powder, and lemon juice, along with vegetables and chicken provide an anti-inflammatory, detoxifying, healing medicine for the body and for the soul.

- 1 tablespoon extra-virgin olive oil
- ½ large yellow onion, chopped
- 1-inch piece fresh ginger, peeled and minced
- 2 teaspoons curry powder
- sea salt and freshly ground black pepper
- 1 cup cooked chicken breast in bite-size pieces
- 3 large kale leaves, stemmed and chopped
- 12 medium cauliflower florets
- 2 medium carrots, peeled and chopped
- 1 celery rib, sliced
- 4 asparagus spears, trimmed and sliced into 1-inch pieces
- ½ small sweet potato, peeled and cut into 1-inch cubes
- 4½ cups low-sodium chicken broth or vegetable broth
- juice of 1 lemon

1. Heat the oil in a medium pot over medium-high heat. After a minute, add the onion and cook, stirring, until the onion softens and begins to color, about 5 minutes.

2. Stir in the ginger and curry powder and season to taste with salt and black pepper. Cook until the ginger is aromatic, about 2 minutes. Add the chicken and vegetables and cook for another 2–3 minutes.

3. Add the broth and turn the heat to high. Once the soup reaches a boil, reduce the heat to low, cover, and simmer until the vegetables are tender, 10–15 minutes.

4. Take the soup off the heat and stir in the lemon juice. Taste for seasoning and add salt and black pepper if needed. Serve hot. Any left-

overs can be stored in the refrigerator for up to 4 days or in the freezer for up to 6 months.

Nutritional analysis per serving (¾ cup): calories 163, fat 6 g, saturated fat 1 g, cholesterol 55 mg, fiber 2 g, protein 20 g, carbohydrate 10 g, sodium 543 mg

SOUTHWESTERN CHICKEN AND VEGETABLE SOUP

Serves: 6

Prep time:
15 minutes

Cook time:
25 minutes

Level: Easy

Budget: $

Smoky and spicy from the paprika and cinnamon, this is not your mom's chicken soup! Enjoy this hearty chicken soup on days when you want something extraordinary and incredibly satisfying.

- 2 tablespoons extra-virgin olive oil
- 1 cup fresh or frozen corn
- 1 large Vidalia onion, chopped
- 1 large green bell pepper, seeded and chopped
- 2 garlic cloves, minced
- 1 teaspoon ground cumin
- 2 teaspoons sweet smoked paprika
- ½ teaspoon ground cinnamon
- 1 (28-ounce) can low-sodium tomato sauce
- 4 cups low-sodium chicken or vegetable broth
- Freshly ground black pepper
- meat from 1 roasted or rotisserie chicken, shredded
- 1 cup water
- 1 avocado, peeled, pitted, and chopped, for garnish

1. Heat the oil in a large pot over medium-high heat. Add the corn and sauté until the kernels are lightly charred around the edges.

2. Add the onion, bell pepper, and garlic and cook until soft, 3–4 minutes. Stir in the cumin, paprika, and cinnamon and sauté for 5 minutes.

3. Add the tomato sauce and broth and season the soup to taste with salt and black pepper. Stir in the shredded chicken and thin the soup with the water.

4. Turn up the heat and bring the soup to a boil. Turn the heat to low and simmer for 10–15 minutes to let the flavors come together. Check for seasoning and adjust if needed with salt or black pepper.

5. Serve the soup garnished with a few pieces of avocado over each portion. Leftover soup can be refrigerated for up to 4 days or frozen for up to 4 months.

Nutritional analysis per serving (1 cup): calories 324, fat 12 g, saturated fat 2 g, cholesterol 81 mg, fiber 57 g, protein 32 g, carbohydrate 24 g, sodium 680 mg

BRANDY'S HEALTHY TURKEY–PINTO BEAN CHILI

Serves: 15

Prep time: 15 minutes

Cook time: 1 hour 20 minutes

Level: Easy

Budget: $$

The chipotle powder in this chili lends a slightly smoky spiciness that invigorates your senses. The combination of beans and turkey make this meal a great source of fiber and protein to stabilize your blood sugar and keep you satisfied for hours.

- 1 tablespoon extra-virgin olive oil
- 3 tablespoons chili powder
- 1 teaspoon ground chipotle chile powder
- 2 teaspoons ground cumin
- 2 teaspoons dried oregano
- 1 large red onion, chopped
- 2 large red bell peppers, seeded and chopped
- 6 garlic cloves, minced
- 2 pounds lean ground turkey
- sea salt and freshly ground black pepper
- 6 cups cooked pinto beans or 3 (15-ounce) cans pinto beans, rinsed and drained
- 1 (28-ounce) can crushed tomatoes
- 1 cup low-sodium chicken broth
- ¼ cup chopped fresh cilantro, for garnish

1. Heat the oil in a large, heavy pot over medium heat. After a minute add the chili powder, chipotle chile powder, cumin, and oregano and toast, stirring, for 30 seconds.

2. Add the onion, bell peppers, and garlic and cook in the spiced oil for 2–3 minutes, stirring frequently.

3. Add the turkey to the pan and break it up as it cooks. Season the turkey to taste with salt and black pepper and cook until brown, 6–8 minutes.

4. Add the beans, tomatoes, and broth and simmer the chili over low heat for 1 hour. Check for seasoning and add salt and black pepper to taste. Garnish the chili with cilantro and serve. Leftover chili can be refrigerated for up to 5 days or frozen for up to 4 months.

Nutritional analysis per serving (1 cup): calories 351, fat 5 g, saturated fat 1 g, cholesterol 33 mg, fiber 13 g, protein 28 g, carbohydrate 20 g, sodium 176 mg

TEXAS-STYLE TURKEY CHILI

Try this nourishing, antioxidant-rich chili the next time you want a hearty and healthy meal on a cool fall or winter night. The aroma from the cocoa and chili powder will make your kitchen come to life, and the flavors will intensify the longer they infuse together.

Serves: 6

Prep time: 15 minutes

Cook time: 1 hour 20 minutes

Level: Easy

Budget: $$

- ¼ cup grapeseed oil
- 1 tablespoon unsweetened cocoa powder
- ¼ cup chili powder
- 1 teaspoon paprika
- 1 teaspoon ground cumin
- 1 teaspoon dried oregano
- 1 large yellow onion, chopped
- 4 garlic cloves, minced
- 1 poblano chile, seeded and finely chopped
- 2 celery ribs, chopped
- 4 large carrots, peeled and chopped
- 2 pounds lean ground turkey
- sea salt and freshly ground black pepper
- 2 cups cooked black beans or 1 (15-ounce) can black beans, rinsed and drained
- 1 (28-ounce) can crushed tomatoes
- 2 tablespoons tomato paste
- 1 cup low-sodium chicken broth

1. Heat the oil in a large, heavy pot over medium heat. After a minute add the cocoa, chili powder, paprika, cumin, and oregano and toast, stirring, for 30 seconds.

2. Add the onion, garlic, poblano, celery, and carrots and cook until soft, 4–5 minutes.

3. Turn the heat to medium-high and add the turkey to the pan. Season the turkey to taste with salt and black pepper and break it up as it cooks. Cook until brown and crumbly, 6–8 minutes.

4. Add the beans, tomatoes, tomato paste, and broth and simmer the chili over low heat for 1 hour. Check for seasoning and add more salt and black pepper if desired. Serve immediately. Leftover chili can be refrigerated for up to 5 days or frozen for up to 3 months.

Nutritional analysis per serving (1 cup): calories 228, fat 8 g, saturated fat 2 g, cholesterol 64 mg, fiber 7 g, protein 23 g, carbohydrate 19 g, sodium 399 mg

SALADS

SUMMER SALAD

Serves: 2

Prep time: 10 minutes

Level: Easy

Budget: $

Summer is a wonderful time to enjoy tomatoes and cucumbers with balsamic vinegar, a little bit of lemon, and a drizzle of extra-virgin olive oil. This is a dish to live for.

DRESSING:

- juice of 1 lemon
- ½ teaspoon balsamic vinegar
- sea salt and freshly ground black pepper
- 2 tablespoons extra-virgin olive oil

SALAD:

- 1 large heirloom tomato, thickly sliced
- 1 avocado, peeled, pitted, and sliced
- 1 large cucumber, chopped

MAKE THE DRESSING:

Combine the lemon juice, balsamic vinegar, and salt and black pepper to taste in a small bowl and whisk to combine. Slowly pour in the olive oil while whisking until the dressing thickens slightly and is emulsified.

ASSEMBLE THE SALAD:

Combine the tomato, avocado, and cucumber in a medium bowl and pour over the dressing. Toss the salad gently to coat all the vegetables evenly and serve.

Nutritional analysis per serving (1 cup): calories 269, fat 22 g, saturated fat 3 g, cholesterol 0 mg, fiber 8 g, protein 4 g, carbohydrate 18 g, sodium 90 mg

BEAN SALAD

Serves: 8

Prep time:
10 minutes

Cook time:
10 minutes

Chill time:
4 hours

Level: Easy

Budget: $

Low-starch beans are a wonderful way to get fiber, protein, and minerals like magnesium into your diet. Combine them with vegetables and lemon to make a healthy, quick, and easy lunch.

- ½ cup extra-virgin olive oil
- 4 garlic cloves, minced
- 4 cups cooked black beans or 2 (15-ounce) cans black beans, rinsed and drained
- 4 celery ribs, thinly sliced
- 1 small red onion, thinly sliced
- ½ cup chopped fresh cilantro
- 2 tablespoons chopped fresh tarragon
- juice of 3 lemons
- zest of 1 lemon
- 1 teaspoon sea salt
- ¼ teaspoon freshly ground black pepper

1. Heat the olive oil in a small pan over low heat. After a minute or two, add the garlic and turn off the heat. Let the garlic sit in the oil for 10 minutes off the heat.

2. Combine all of the ingredients, including the garlic-infused olive oil, in a large bowl and mix well.

3. Refrigerate for at least 4 hours and serve cold. Store any leftover bean salad in the refrigerator for up to 4 days.

Nutritional analysis per serving (¾ cup): calories 250, fat 14 g, saturated fat 2 g, cholesterol 0 mg, fiber 9 g, protein 8 g, carbohydrate 25 g, sodium 467 mg

CHICKPEA AND KALE SALAD

This quick and easy recipe is also affordable, healthy, and simply delicious.

Serves: 3

Prep time:
5 minutes

Level: Easy

Budget: $

DRESSING:

- juice of ½ large lemon
- 2 tablespoons extra-virgin olive oil
- sea salt and freshly ground black pepper

SALAD:

- 2 cups cooked chickpeas or 1 (15-ounce) can chickpeas, rinsed and drained
- 3 large kale leaves, stemmed and cut into 2-inch pieces
- 1 large red bell pepper, seeded and chopped
- 3 scallions, thinly sliced

MAKE THE DRESSING:

In a small bowl whisk together the lemon juice and olive oil and season to taste with salt and black pepper.

ASSEMBLE THE SALAD:

In a medium bowl combine the chickpeas, kale, bell pepper, and scallions. Pour the dressing over the vegetables and toss until evenly coated. Serve.

Nutritional analysis per serving (1 cup): calories 230, fat 10 g, saturated fat 1 g, cholesterol 0 mg, fiber 6 g, protein 8 g, carbohydrate 25 g, sodium 348 mg

CARIBBEAN BLACK-EYED PEA SALAD

Serves: 4

Prep time:
10 minutes

Level: Easy

Budget: $

This salad is a dynamic mixture of fresh cilantro, garlic, lemon, and peppers that naturally blend together to create a delicious plant-based lunch.

DRESSING:

- ¾ cup low-sodium vegetable broth
- 1 garlic clove, minced
- 2 tablespoons lemon juice
- 3 tablespoons chopped fresh cilantro
- ¼ teaspoon chopped fresh oregano
- ¼ teaspoon cayenne pepper
- ⅛ teaspoon red pepper flakes
- ½ teaspoon sea salt
- 1 tablespoon extra-virgin olive oil

SALAD:

- 4 cups cooked black-eyed peas or 2 (15-ounce) cans black-eyed peas, drained and rinsed
- ½ large poblano pepper, diced
- 7 scallions (white part only), finely chopped
- ½ large red onion, minced

MAKE THE DRESSING:

In a small bowl combine the vegetable broth, garlic, lemon juice, cilantro, oregano, cayenne pepper, red pepper flakes, and salt in a medium bowl. Slowly whisk in the olive oil until the dressing thickens slightly and emulsifies.

ASSEMBLE THE SALAD:

In a large salad bowl, gently mix the beans, pepper, scallions, and onion. Pour the dressing over the beans and vegetables and toss until everything is evenly dressed. Serve. Leftover black-eyed pea salad can be refrigerated for up to 4 days.

Nutritional analysis per serving (1 cup): calories 178, fat 4 g, saturated fat 0 g, cholesterol 0 mg, fiber 7 g, protein 10 g, carbohydrate 28 g, sodium 322 mg

RED CABBAGE SALAD

Serves: 2

Prep time:
15 minutes

Chill time:
1 hour

Level: Easy

Budget: $

In this citrus–scented salad, the orange and coriander marry well together. Try this refreshing salad the next time you want to expand your repertoire of preparing cruciferous vegetables.

- 1 cup shredded red cabbage
- 1 tablespoon extra-virgin olive oil
- 1 tablespoon balsamic vinegar
- 1 tablespoon apple cider vinegar
- zest of ½ large orange
- ½ teaspoon ground coriander
- sea salt and freshly ground black pepper
- ¼ cup chopped fresh cilantro

1. Combine the cabbage, olive oil, vinegars, and orange zest in a large bowl.
2. Add the coriander and season to taste with salt and black pepper. Toss until well mixed.
3. Refrigerate for 1 hour, then add the cilantro. Serve chilled.

Nutritional analysis per serving (1 cup): calories 73, fat 7 g, saturated fat 1 g, cholesterol 0 mg, fiber 1 g, protein 1 g, carbohydrate 2 g, sodium 125 mg

BLACK BEAN TOFU SALAD

Tofu contains isoflavones, plant compounds that may help balance women's health. The lean protein from tofu coupled with the healthy fat from the walnut oil make this salad a wonderful addition to your anti-inflammatory lifestyle.

Serves: 4

Prep time: 10 minutes

Chill time: 2 hours

Level: Easy

Budget: $

DRESSING:

- ⅓ cup apple cider vinegar
- 2 garlic cloves, minced
- ½ teaspoon dried herb or seasoning blend of choice
- 3 tablespoons walnut oil
- sea salt and freshly ground black pepper

SALAD:

- 2 cups cooked black beans or 1 (15-ounce) can black beans, rinsed and drained
- 6 ounces firm tofu, drained, pressed, and crumbled
- 2 celery ribs, chopped
- ½ medium red onion, chopped
- ½ large red bell pepper, seeded and chopped
- ½ large yellow bell pepper, seeded and chopped
- 1 medium carrot, peeled and shredded
- ¼ cup chopped fresh cilantro leaves
- 1 large head Bibb lettuce

MAKE THE DRESSING:

Combine the vinegar, garlic, and herbs in a blender. Blend on medium speed and slowly pour in the oil. Season to taste with salt and black pepper and blend for 2 minutes until well mixed and emulsified.

ASSEMBLE THE SALAD:

In a large bowl combine all of the salad ingredients except the lettuce, and stir until well mixed. Pour most of the dressing over the salad and gently toss until well coated. Taste and add more dressing until as dressed as you desire. Refrigerate for 2 hours and serve each portion over 2–3 lettuce leaves. Any leftovers can be refrigerated for up to 4 days.

Nutritional analysis per serving (1½ cups): calories 191, fat 6 g, saturated fat 1 g, cholesterol 0 mg, fiber 8 g, protein 12 g, carbohydrate 23 g, sodium 45 mg

SHRIMP AND AVOCADO SALAD

This fast, simple salad is a delicious and refreshing way to enjoy shrimp for lunch or dinner. The flavors of mango, lime, and sesame give it a sweet, tangy, delectable taste.

Serves: 2
Prep time: 15 minutes
Level: Moderate
Budget: $$

- 8 ounces frozen cooked shrimp, thawed
- 1 cup cherry tomatoes, halved
- 1 garlic clove, minced
- 1 mango, peeled, pitted, and diced
- 1 avocado, peeled, pitted, and diced
- juice of 1 lime
- 1 tablespoon toasted sesame oil
- 1 tablespoon sesame seeds
- 1 tablespoon chopped fresh cilantro
- pinch of red pepper flakes
- 2 cups chopped Boston or romaine lettuce

In a medium bowl, combine all of the ingredients except for the lettuce. Toss well. Arrange the lettuce on two salad plates. Top with the shrimp and avocado salad and serve.

Nutritional analysis per serving (2 cups): calories 303, fat 11 g, saturated fat 2 g, cholesterol 224 mg, fiber 4 g, protein 27 g, carbohydrate 28 g, sodium 270 mg

Serves: 4

Prep time:
20 minutes

Cook time:
15 minutes

Level: Easy

Budget: $

ENTRÉES

QUINOA-BEAN-VEGETABLE CUTLETS WITH BEAN SPROUTS AND CILANTRO CHUTNEY

The turmeric in these vegetarian cutlets is just one of the many magical ingredients that make this a remarkable, anti-inflammatory meal. These cutlets are a creative way to explore Indian cooking. Be sure to make the cilantro chutney to add extra zing.

CUTLETS:

- ¼ cup cooked quinoa
- ½ cup cooked kidney beans or ¼ (15-ounce) can, rinsed and drained
- ½ cup cooked yellow lentils
- 1 tablespoon grapeseed oil, plus ¼ cup for frying
- 1 teaspoon cumin seeds
- ½ teaspoon ground turmeric
- 1 small red onion, finely chopped
- 1-inch piece fresh ginger, peeled and grated
- 1 serrano pepper, seeded and finely chopped
- sea salt and freshly ground black pepper
- 2 large kale leaves, stemmed and finely chopped
- ½ small head broccoli, finely chopped
- 1 medium red bell pepper, seeded and finely chopped
- ½ cup garbanzo bean flour
- 2 cups mung bean sprouts

CILANTRO CHUTNEY:

- 1 bunch (about 3 ounces) cilantro, stems removed
- 2 tablespoons roasted peanuts
- 1-inch piece fresh ginger, peeled and coarsely chopped
- juice of ½ lime

MAKE THE CUTLETS:

1. Combine the quinoa, beans, and lentils in a medium bowl and set aside.

2. Heat 1 tablespoon of the oil in a large cast-iron pan over medium heat. When the oil is hot, toast the cumin and turmeric until the cumin begins to pop. Immediately add the onion, ginger, and serrano pepper and cook, stirring, until the onions begin to brown, 5–6 minutes. Season the mixture with a large pinch of salt and black pepper, and add the kale, broccoli, and bell pepper. Cook, stirring, until the vegetables soften slightly, 2–3 minutes. Turn off the heat.

3. Add the onion and kale mixture to the bowl with the quinoa and beans, and mash them together using a large fork. Once the mixture is smooth, check it for seasoning and add additional salt or black pepper if desired.

4. Put the garbanzo bean flour on a small plate. Form the bean mixture into 4 equal patties and dredge them in flour on both sides.

5. Heat the cast-iron pan again over medium heat and add the remaining ¼ cup oil. Shallow-fry the cutlets until brown and crisp, 3–4 minutes per side. Let the cutlets rest while you make the chutney.

MAKE THE CHUTNEY:

Combine all of the chutney ingredients in a food processor and pulse until smooth but thick.

ASSEMBLE THE CUTLETS:

Place a large handful of bean sprouts on each plate, lay a cutlet on top of the sprouts, and top each portion with cilantro chutney. Serve immediately. Uncooked cutlets and leftover chutney can be stored in the refrigerator for up to 4 days.

Nutritional analysis per serving (1 cutlet): calories 175, fat 8 g, saturated fat 1 g, cholesterol 0 mg, fiber 7 g, protein 6 g, carbohydrate 21 g, sodium 604 mg

CHINESE FRIED QUINOA

Serves: 4

Prep time:
15 minutes

Cook time:
25 minutes

Level: Easy

Budget: $

This is a simple stir-fry to prepare anytime you want something fragrant and delicious to permeate the walls of your home. The broccoli contributes cancer-fighting glucosinolates and the chili flakes give your metabolism a boost.

SAUCE:

- 1 tablespoon reduced-sodium, gluten-free tamari
- 2 teaspoons toasted sesame oil
- juice of 1 lime
- sea salt and freshly ground black pepper to taste
- red pepper flakes to taste

STIR-FRY:

- 1 tablespoon peanut oil
- 1 medium white onion, chopped
- 2 garlic cloves, minced
- 1-inch piece fresh ginger, peeled and finely grated
- ½ small head broccoli, cut into small florets
- 1 large carrot, peeled and cut into matchsticks
- 2 celery ribs, thinly sliced
- 1 large red bell pepper, seeded and thinly sliced
- 1 cup fresh or frozen peas
- 2 cups cooked quinoa

MAKE THE SAUCE:

In a small bowl whisk together all of the sauce ingredients. Set aside.

MAKE THE STIR-FRY:

1. Heat the oil in a large wok over medium-high heat. Add the onion, garlic, and ginger to the hot oil and stir-fry until soft and fragrant, 1–2 minutes.

2. Stir in the broccoli and stir-fry until it turns a brighter shade of green, 2–3 minutes.

3. Add the carrots, celery, bell pepper, and peas and stir-fry until the vegetables have softened, 3–4 minutes.

4. Once the broccoli is tender, turn the heat to high and add the quinoa and reserved sauce. Toss the vegetables and the quinoa until they are evenly mixed and the quinoa is slightly crispy. Check for seasoning and add more tamari, salt, and black pepper if desired.

5. Transfer to a platter and serve alongside your protein of choice. Any leftovers can be refrigerated for up to 4 days.

Nutritional analysis per serving (1 cup): calories 227, fat 8 g, saturated fat 1 g, cholesterol 0 mg, fiber 8 g, protein 8 g, carbohydrate 33 g, sodium 429 mg

WHITE BEANS ON A BED OF GREENS

Serves: 4

Prep time:
10 minutes

Level: Easy

Budget: $

If you are looking for a quick lunch to satisfy your hunger and promote stable blood sugar throughout the afternoon, this dish is perfect for you.

- 2 cups cooked cannellini beans or 1 (15-ounce) can cannellini beans, rinsed and drained
- juice of 1 lemon
- ½ cup chopped fresh parsley
- 1 garlic clove, minced
- 2 tablespoons extra-virgin olive oil
- sea salt and freshly ground black pepper to taste
- 6 cups fresh mixed baby greens

1. In a medium bowl, mix all of the ingredients except the baby greens.
2. Divide the greens among four plates and serve the white bean salad on top. Any leftover bean salad can be stored in the refrigerator, separate from the salad greens, for up to 4 days.

Nutritional analysis per serving (½ cup): calories 228, fat 7 g, saturated fat 2 g, cholesterol 0 mg, fiber 7 g, protein 11 g, carbohydrate 32 g, sodium 56 mg

CURRIED SPINACH WITH CHICKPEAS AND COCONUT MILK

Coconut milk is a creamy, delicious addition to your diet. This recipe features chickpeas, but you could add any beans or vegetables—use your imagination!

- ½ cup extra-virgin olive oil
- 4 medium Vidalia onions, finely chopped
- ¼ cup curry powder
- 3 tablespoons garlic powder
- ½ teaspoon cayenne pepper
- 1½ pounds spinach, chopped
- 10 cups cooked chickpeas or 5 (15-ounce) cans, rinsed and drained
- 5 (13.5-ounce) cans unsweetened coconut milk

Serves: 10
Prep time: 10 minutes
Cook time: 20 minutes
Level: Easy
Budget: $

1. Heat the oil in a large cast-iron pan over medium-high heat. Add the onions and sauté until brown, 8–10 minutes.
2. Stir in the curry powder, garlic powder, and cayenne pepper and cook for an additional minute.
3. Add the spinach to the pan and cook until it wilts, about 5 minutes.
4. Stir in the chickpeas and coconut milk and cook until the chickpeas are warmed through, about 5 minutes. Serve as a side dish or over quinoa as a main dish. Store any leftovers in the refrigerator for up to 5 days.

Nutritional analysis per serving (2 cups): calories 206, fat 13 g, saturated fat 2 g, cholesterol 0 mg, fiber 5 g, protein 7 g, carbohydrate 19 g, sodium 56 mg

SAUTÉED SPINACH AND TOMATOES OVER ROASTED SPAGHETTI SQUASH

Serves: 4

Prep time:
10 minutes

Cook time:
1 hour

Level:
Moderate

Budget: $

Spaghetti squash is a fun vegetable. It is crunchy and pasta-like and, with spinach, tomatoes, and pine nuts, makes a wonderful, simple meal.

- 1 tablespoon extra-virgin olive oil
- 1 large spaghetti squash, halved and seeded
- sea salt and freshly ground black pepper
- ½ cup pine nuts
- 8 garlic cloves, finely chopped
- 1 pound grape tomatoes, halved
- 8 ounces baby spinach
- 10 fresh basil leaves, finely sliced

1. Preheat the oven to 350°F.

2. Brush the cut sides of the squash with 1 teaspoon of the oil and season generously with salt and black pepper. Place the squash, cut sides down, on a baking sheet and roast for 30–40 minutes. The squash is cooked when a knife easily pierces through the skin and flesh. Let cool enough to handle, shred the flesh with a fork into spaghetti-like threads, and set aside.

3. Turn the oven up to 400°F.

4. Spread the pine nuts on a small baking sheet and toast them until golden brown, 3–5 minutes, checking often to make sure they don't get too dark.

5. Heat the remaining 2 teaspoons oil in a large sauté pan over medium heat. After a minute add the garlic to the pan and cook, stirring constantly, for 2–3 minutes.

6. Add the tomatoes, season to taste with salt and black pepper, and cook until the tomatoes begin to burst, 5–6 minutes.

7. Add the spinach to the pan and season to taste with salt and black pepper. Cook, stirring, until the spinach just wilts, 3–4 minutes.

8. Divide the spaghetti squash among 4 plates, and top with the sautéed spinach and tomatoes. Sprinkle on the roasted pine nuts and fresh basil. Serve immediately. Any leftovers can be refrigerated for up to 4 days.

Nutritional analysis per serving (2 cups): calories 254, fat 17 g, saturated fat 2 g, cholesterol 0 mg, fiber 5 g, protein 8 g, carbohydrate 25 g, sodium 128 mg

ASIAN LETTUCE BOATS

Serves: 6

Prep time:
15 minutes

Cook time:
15 minutes

Level: Easy

Budget: $

These hearty vegetarian lettuce boats are slightly sweet, full of healthy vegetables, and mixed with just the right amount of sesame-peanut sauce to add depth to the meal. Sprinkle some fresh cilantro on top before serving to make the flavors pop.

- ¾ cup walnuts
- 2 tablespoons grapeseed oil
- 1 medium red bell pepper, seeded and finely chopped
- 2 scallions, finely sliced
- 1 large kale leaf, stemmed and finely chopped
- 1 teaspoon toasted sesame oil
- 2 tablespoons reduced-sodium, gluten-free tamari
- 1 tablespoon peanut satay sauce
- 1 tablespoon orange juice
- sea salt and freshly ground black pepper
- 6 large Bibb lettuce leaves
- 3 tablespoons chopped fresh cilantro

1. Pulse the walnuts in a food processor until finely chopped. Drizzle 1 tablespoon of the grapeseed oil in toward the end of grinding to moisten the walnuts; the consistency should look like ground meat when done.

2. Heat the remaining 1 tablespoon oil in a medium cast-iron pan. After a minute add the bell pepper, scallions, and kale. Cook until the pepper is soft and the kale wilts, 3–4 minutes.

3. Add the sesame oil, tamari, peanut satay sauce, and orange juice. Stir until well mixed.

4. Add the walnut mixture, stir to combine, and season to taste with salt and black pepper.

5. Turn off the heat and let the mixture cool briefly. Spoon the filling into individual lettuce leaves and garnish with the cilantro and serve

immediately. If not eating right away, store the walnut mixture in the refrigerator, separate from the lettuce. Fill the boats right before serving so the lettuce stays crisp. Any leftover filling can be refrigerated for up to 4 days.

Nutritional analysis per serving (1 lettuce boat): calories 176, fat 16 g, saturated fat 2 g, cholesterol 0 mg, fiber 2 g, protein 6 g, carbohydrate 6 g, sodium 337 mg

SWEET POTATO BURGERS

Serves: 8

Prep time:
20 minutes

Cook time:
55 minutes

Level: Easy

Budget: $

Almond flour, beans, and sweet potatoes together create a low-glycemic yet delicious burger, which can be enjoyed with a salad.

SWEET POTATO BURGERS:

- 1 large sweet potato
- 1 tablespoon plus 1 teaspoon extra-virgin olive oil
- sea salt and freshly ground black pepper
- 4 cups cooked cannellini beans or 2 (15-ounce) cans cannellini beans, rinsed and drained
- 2 teaspoons favorite spice blend, such as Cajun or curry powder
- ¼ teaspoon cayenne pepper
- ¼ cup almond flour
- 5 ounces mixed salad greens
- 1 avocado, peeled, pitted, and sliced

TAHINI DRESSING:

- 2 tablespoons tahini paste
- juice and zest of 1 large lemon
- 1 garlic clove, minced

MAKE THE BURGERS:

1. Preheat the oven to 400°F. Line a small baking sheet with foil.

2. Using a fork, prick deep holes all over the sweet potato. Brush it with 1 teaspoon of the olive oil. Season generously with salt and black pepper and bake until completely soft, 45–50 minutes; a knife should easily slide through. Let it cool until you can handle it.

3. Peel the sweet potato and place the flesh in a medium bowl. Add the beans and mash the potato and beans together with a potato masher or large fork. Season the mixture with the spice blend, cayenne pepper, and salt and black pepper to taste.

4. Stir in the almond flour and shape the mixture into 8 patties.

5. Heat the remaining 1 tablespoon oil in a large cast-iron pan and brown the patties until crispy and golden brown, 3–4 minutes per side.

MAKE THE DRESSING:

In a small bowl whisk together all of the dressing ingredients until smooth. Season to taste with salt and black pepper.

ASSEMBLE THE BURGERS:

Place the burgers on a bed of greens and top each one with a few slices of avocado. Drizzle a little tahini dressing over each burger and serve immediately. You may also add your favorite burger toppings such as caramelized onions, sautéed mushrooms, or your favorite burger condiment. Any leftover sweet potato mixture can be refrigerated for up to 4 days.

Nutritional analysis per serving (1 burger): calories 143, fat 5 g, saturated fat 0 g, cholesterol 0 mg, fiber 6 g, protein 7 g, carbohydrate 20 g, sodium 192 mg

SHIRATAKI NOODLES WITH KALE AND CHICKPEAS

Serves: 4

Prep time:
5 minutes

Cook time:
15 minutes

Level: Easy

Budget: $

You can enjoy "pasta" in this tasty, light, and nutrient-rich comfort meal. These plant-based noodles explode with fiber from the konjac root, and shiitake mushrooms boast immune-boosting properties to help keep you healthy and feeling great.

- 2 tablespoons extra-virgin olive oil
- 3 garlic cloves, minced
- 1 large bunch kale, stemmed and roughly chopped
- 2 cups cooked chickpeas or 1 (15-ounce) can chickpeas, rinsed and drained
- 2 (8-ounce) packages shirataki noodles, drained
- 4 ounces shiitake mushrooms, stemmed and thickly sliced
- ½ cup marinara sauce
- sea salt and freshly ground black pepper
- ¼ cup chopped fresh parsley, for garnish

1. Heat the oil in a medium cast-iron pan over medium heat. Add the garlic and cook, stirring, until aromatic, about 1 minute.

2. Toss in the kale and sauté it in the garlic oil until it wilts, 3–4 minutes.

3. Add the chickpeas, noodles, shiitakes, and marinara sauce and warm through for 3 minutes. Season to taste with salt and black pepper. Transfer to a platter, garnish with parsley, and serve. Any leftover noodles can be refrigerated for up to 3 days.

Nutritional analysis per serving (1½ cups): calories 215, fat 10 g, saturated fat 1 g, cholesterol 0 mg, fiber 8 g, protein 9 g, carbohydrate 25 g, sodium 155 mg

END-OF-THE-GARDEN ZUCCHINI MEAL

Tomatoes, bell peppers, and jalapeños provide a wealth of antioxidants. Enjoy this dish at the peak of summer to reap the most flavor from the zucchini and corn. It will cool you down with its delightful array of fresh herbs and aromatics.

Serves: 6

Prep time: 15 minutes

Cook time: 40 minutes

Level: Easy

Budget: $

QUINOA:

- 1 cup uncooked quinoa
- 1 cup water
- ½ teaspoon sea salt

ZUCCHINI:

- 1 tablespoon grapeseed oil
- 1½ pounds lean ground beef
- sea salt and freshly ground black pepper
- 1 large yellow onion, chopped
- 1 large green bell pepper, seeded and chopped
- 1 medium jalapeño pepper, seeded and minced
- 2 garlic cloves, minced
- 2 teaspoons chili powder
- ¼ cup chopped fresh cilantro
- 5 medium zucchini, chopped
- 2 large tomatoes, chopped
- 1¼ cups fresh or frozen corn
- 1 (15-ounce) can diced tomatoes with green chilies, undrained

MAKE THE QUINOA:

1. Dry-toast the quinoa in a medium pot over medium-high heat until aromatic, 3–4 minutes.
2. Add the water and salt and bring to a boil. Cover the pan, reduce the heat to low, and simmer until all of the liquid has evaporated and the quinoa is cooked, about 25 minutes.

3. Turn off the heat and let the quinoa steam in the covered pot for 3–5 minutes.

4. Fluff the quinoa with a fork and transfer to a large bowl.

MAKE THE ZUCCHINI:

1. Heat the oil in a wide cast-iron pan over medium-high heat and add the beef. Season to taste with salt and black pepper and break up the meat as it browns, about 3-5 minutes.

2. Add the onion, bell pepper, jalapeño, and garlic and cook until the vegetables are soft, 5–6 minutes.

3. Add the remaining ingredients and cover the pan. Reduce the heat to low and simmer until the zucchini are tender, 20–25 minutes. Serve the zucchini mixture over the quinoa. Any leftover zucchini can be refrigerated for up to 4 days.

Nutritional analysis per serving (1½ cups): calories 271, fat 11 g, saturated fat 5 g, cholesterol 75 mg, fiber 4 g, protein 26 g, carbohydrate 15 g, sodium 402 mg

Spaghetti Squash Pad Thai

In this classic Thai dish you can maximize your nutrition by trading carbohydrate-rich rice noodles for low-glycemic and vitamin-A-rich spaghetti squash. You'll find Thai fish sauce in your local Asian or natural foods market, or in the international aisle of most large supermarkets.

- 1 large spaghetti squash, halved and seeded
- ¼ cup peanut oil
- 1 tablespoon Thai fish sauce
- 2 teaspoons reduced-sodium, gluten-free tamari sauce
- ½ teaspoon red pepper flakes
- 1 large egg, beaten
- 2 garlic cloves, minced
- 4 ounces boneless, skinless chicken breasts, roughly chopped
- sea salt
- 4 ounces raw shrimp, peeled, deveined, and roughly chopped
- 2 large carrots, peeled and shredded
- 2 cups mung bean sprouts
- 6 scallions, finely chopped
- 1 lime, halved
- ¼ cup chopped roasted peanuts, for garnish

Serves: 4	
Prep time: 15 minutes	
Cook time: 40 minutes	
Level: Easy	
Budget: $	

1. Preheat the oven to 400°F.
2. Brush the cut sides of the squash with 1 tablespoon of the peanut oil. Place the squash, cut sides down, on a baking sheet and roast for 30–40 minutes. The squash is cooked when a knife easily pierces through the skin and flesh. Let cool, use a fork to shred the flesh into spaghetti-like strands, and set aside.
3. In a small bowl stir together the fish sauce, tamari, and red pepper flakes. Set aside.

4. Heat 1 tablespoon of the oil in a large wok or large cast-iron pan over medium-high heat. Add the egg and cook until scrambled, 30–60 seconds, breaking it up. Transfer to a plate and reserve.

5. Pour another tablespoon of the oil into the wok and stir-fry the garlic until aromatic. Season the chicken with a little salt and add it to the pan. Stir-fry the chicken until golden brown, about 4 minutes. Push the chicken to the side and add the shrimp in the center of the pan. Stir frequently until the shrimp are pink and firm, about 3 minutes.

6. Toss in the carrots and stir-fry them for 1 minute. Transfer the contents of the pan to a platter.

7. Add the remaining 1 tablespoon oil to the wok, spread the squash strands out in the pan, and cook for 1 minute without stirring. Flip the pile of strands over and brown them for 2 minutes on the other side.

8. Pour the sauce into the wok and add the chicken-shrimp mixture, egg, bean sprouts, and scallions. Gently toss to heat through, and squeeze the juice of one lime half over all. Garnish with the peanuts and serve with the other half lime available for table-side squeezing. Any leftovers can be refrigerated for up to 4 days.

Nutritional analysis per serving (1⅓ cups): calories 263, fat 15 g, saturated fat 2 g, cholesterol 131 mg, fiber 1 g, protein 21 g, carbohydrate 14 g, sodium 611 mg

Coconut Shrimp with Lemongrass Quinoa and Thai Vegetables

Serves: 2

Prep time: 15 minutes

Cook time: 30 minutes

Level: Moderate

Budget: $$

Lemongrass is the star of this dish, lending a subtle, lemony essence. Lemongrass is used in traditional Thai cuisine and is thought to have immune-boosting properties. Discard everything but the white inner stalk, which is the edible part of the plant.

- ⅓ cup uncooked quinoa
- 1 cup brewed green tea (3 green tea bags steeped in 8 ounces boiling water)
- 1 teaspoon finely chopped lemongrass (inner white stalk only)
- 1 tablespoon extra-virgin coconut oil
- 8 ounces raw shrimp, peeled and deveined
- ½ cup unsweetened coconut milk
- 1 teaspoon ground coriander
- 1 teaspoon finely grated fresh ginger
- 1 teaspoon ground turmeric
- sea salt
- 1 (12-ounce) package frozen Thai-style stir-fry vegetables
- 2 tablespoons chopped fresh cilantro, for garnish

1. Combine the quinoa, green tea, and lemongrass in a small saucepan and bring to a boil over high heat. Reduce the heat, cover, and simmer for 15–20 minutes, until fluffy. Remove the pan from the heat and set aside.

2. Heat the coconut oil in a medium saucepan over medium-high heat. Swirl the oil until the pan is evenly coated. Add the shrimp in one layer and cook on one side for 3 minutes. Carefully turn the shrimp over and cook for another minute. Add the coconut milk, coriander, ginger, turmeric, and sea salt to taste, and stir well. Simmer until the sauce thickens and the shrimp is cooked through, about 2 more minutes.

3. Meanwhile, cook the Thai vegetables according to the package directions.

4. Place 1 cup of quinoa on each plate. Spoon the shrimp and sauce on top. Sprinkle with chopped cilantro. Serve the vegetables on the side. Any leftovers can be refrigerated for up to 3 days.

Nutritional analysis per serving (1 cup shrimp with sauce, 2 cups vegetables): calories 458, fat 22 g, saturated fat 12 g, cholesterol 194 mg, fiber 10 g, protein 36 g, carbohydrate 43 g, sodium 328 mg

ASIAN PRAWN PAELLA

Replace the white rice traditionally used in paella with brown rice, and substitute turmeric for the saffron to lend that beautiful yellow color. The curcumin from the turmeric is an added bonus that not only provides a luxurious bright hue but also doubles as an inflammation-busting antioxidant.

Serves: 2

Prep time:
5 minutes

Cook time:
20 minutes

Level:
Moderate

Budget: $$

- 2 tablespoons grapeseed oil
- 1 tablespoon peanut oil
- 1 medium Vidalia onion, chopped
- 1 large carrot, peeled and chopped
- 3 garlic cloves, minced
- sea salt
- 1 large egg, beaten
- 8 ounces raw shrimp, peeled and deveined
- 2 cups cooked medium-grain brown rice
- 6 scallions, finely sliced
- 3 tablespoons reduced-sodium, gluten-free tamari
- 1 tablespoon ground turmeric
- ¼ cup unsalted cashews, chopped
- 3 tablespoons currants

1. Heat the grapeseed oil and peanut oil in a wok over high heat. Add the onion and carrot and stir-fry until soft, 3–4 minutes.

2. Stir in the garlic, season to taste with salt, and cook until aromatic, 2–3 minutes.

3. Pour in the egg and scramble it quickly and thoroughly (30–60 seconds), breaking it up.

4. Toss in the shrimp and cook until pink and firm, 3–4 minutes.

5. Add the brown rice, scallions, and tamari and toss the rice until fried and light brown.

6. Add the turmeric, cashews, and currants and toss to combine. Reduce the heat to medium-low and continue to stir-fry for 3 more minutes.

7. Remove from the heat, transfer the contents of the wok to a large dish, and serve. Any leftovers can be refrigerated for up to 3 days.

Nutritional analysis per serving (1 cup): calories 335, fat 13 g, saturated fat 3 g, cholesterol 210 mg, fiber 4 g, protein 23 g, carbohydrate 32 g, sodium 525 mg

CITRUS CRAB SALAD

Serves: 2

Prep time: 20 minutes

Level: Easy

Budget: $

Crab is low in saturated fat but a good source of iron, vitamin B_{12}, zinc, copper, and selenium, all of which reduce inflammation. Sunflower sprouts are simply baby sunflower plants and can be found in the produce department. They add a nutritious crunch to salads, wraps, and even soups.

DRESSING:

- 1 tablespoon Dijon mustard
- zest of 1 small orange
- 1 tablespoon extra-virgin olive oil
- 2 tablespoons rice vinegar
- 1 tablespoon chopped fresh dill

SALAD:

- 2 cups shredded red cabbage
- 2 romaine lettuce leaves, chopped
- 1 cup sunflower sprouts
- 1 small red onion, finely sliced
- 1 large orange, peeled and segmented
- 1 (6-ounce) can snow crabmeat

MAKE THE DRESSING:

In a small bowl, whisk the dressing ingredients until well mixed. Set aside.

ASSEMBLE THE SALAD:

In a large bowl, combine the cabbage, lettuce, sprouts, onion, and orange sections. Add the crabmeat and toss gently until combined. Pour the dressing over the crab and vegetable mixture and toss until the salad is evenly coated. Serve immediately.

Nutritional analysis per serving (3 ounces crab, 2 cups salad): calories 265, fat 8 g, saturated fat 1 g, cholesterol 65 mg, fiber 7 g, protein 24 g, carbohydrate 27 g, sodium 389 mg

SWEET AND SOUR COD WITH VEGETABLES AND HERBED QUINOA

Serves: 4

Prep time:
20 minutes

Cook time:
15 minutes

Level:
Moderate

Budget: $$

This dish is as colorful as it is flavorful and healthy. Green tea is not just for drinking! Cook your grains in this antioxidant-rich plant to impart phytonutrients to your meals.

QUINOA:

- ⅓ cup uncooked quinoa
- 1 cup brewed green tea (3 green tea bags steeped in 8 ounces boiling water)
- 1 stalk lemongrass (inner white stalk only), finely chopped

SAUCE:

- 3 tablespoons reduced-sodium, gluten-free tamari
- ¼ cup rice vinegar
- 1-inch piece fresh ginger, peeled and grated
- 3 tablespoons low-sodium ketchup
- 2 teaspoons arrowroot

COD:

- 1 tablespoon extra-virgin olive oil
- 1 medium onion, sliced
- 3 garlic cloves, minced
- 1 pound cod fillets, cut into 1-inch pieces
- 2 cups broccoli florets
- 1 large carrot, peeled and cut into matchsticks
- 2 tablespoons sesame seeds
- 2 tablespoons chopped fresh cilantro, for garnish

MAKE THE QUINOA:

Combine the quinoa, green tea, and lemongrass in a small saucepan and bring to a boil over high heat. Reduce the heat, cover, and simmer for 15–20 minutes. Remove the pan from the heat and set aside.

MAKE THE SAUCE:

Mix together the tamari, vinegar, 1 tablespoon of the ginger, ketchup, and arrowroot in a small saucepan and bring to a boil, stirring constantly. Simmer over high heat until the sauce boils and thickens, about 4 minutes. Remove from the heat and set aside.

MAKE THE COD:

1. Heat the olive oil in a wok or large cast-iron pan over medium heat and sauté the onion, stirring constantly. Add the garlic, remaining ginger, and cod and stir-fry for 2–3 minutes. Add the broccoli and carrots, and continue to stir-fry for another 2–3 minutes, stirring constantly.

2. Add the sauce and sesame seeds and cook until the sauce reduces slightly, about 2 minutes. Serve the cod and vegetables with the steamed quinoa and garnish with chopped cilantro. Any leftovers can be refrigerated for up to 3 days.

Nutritional analysis per serving (4 ounces cod, ¾ cup vegetables): calories 357, fat 8 g, saturated fat 1 g, cholesterol 41 mg, fiber 5 g, protein 29 g, carbohydrate 42 g, sodium 574 mg

WILD RICE AND SALMON WITH COLLARDS

Serves: 2

Prep time:
20 minutes

Cook time:
1 hour

Level: Easy

Budget: $

Dill and lemon are a refreshing addition to the salmon. Toasting the sesame seeds and rice brings out a subtle nutty flavor, which perfumes this dish. Everyone will congregate in the kitchen to soak in the aromas.

- ½ cup uncooked wild rice
- 2 (3-ounce) skin-on salmon fillets
- 2 teaspoons sesame oil
- 3 teaspoons chopped fresh dill
- sea salt and freshly ground black pepper
- ½ small lemon
- 1 teaspoon extra-virgin coconut oil
- 1 tablespoon black sesame seeds
- 2 cups low-sodium vegetable broth
- 2 cups cooked chickpeas or 1 (15-ounce) can chickpeas, rinsed and drained
- 2 garlic cloves, minced
- 1 large head red collard greens, stemmed and roughly chopped
- 10 fresh cilantro leaves

1. Soak the rice for 2–3 hours in enough fresh water to cover by two inches. Drain well and set aside.

2. Preheat the oven to 400°F.

3. Lay the salmon fillets on a cutting board and brush them with 1 teaspoon of the sesame oil. Season both sides with the dill and salt and black pepper to taste, and squeeze lemon juice over them. Let them sit while you prepare the rice.

4. Heat the coconut oil in a small pot over medium–high heat. Add the rice and sesame seeds and toast, stirring constantly, for 3–5 minutes. Pour in 1½ cups of the broth and add a pinch of salt to the rice. Reduce the heat to low, cover, and simmer until the rice absorbs all of the liquid, 50-55 minutes. Just before the rice is finished cooking, add the chickpeas. Put the cover back on and let the chickpeas steam briefly to warm up.

5. After allowing the salmon to marinate for a few minutes, place it on a lightly greased baking sheet and bake until cooked through, 8–10 minutes.

6. While the salmon is cooking, heat the remaining 1 teaspoon sesame oil in a medium pot over medium heat. Add the garlic and cook for about a minute. Pour in the remaining vegetable broth and add the collard greens. Cook until the leaves wilt, about 3 minutes.

7. To serve, lay down a bed of rice and collards on each plate and place the salmon on top. Garnish with a few leaves of cilantro and serve hot. Any leftovers can be refrigerated for up to 3 days.

Nutritional analysis per serving (½ recipe): calories 457, fat 21 g, saturated fat 5 g, cholesterol 54 mg, fiber 10 g, protein 30 g, carbohydrate 39 g, sodium 313 mg

Wild Salmon with Rosemary Sweet Potatoes and Lemon Asparagus

Serves: 2

Prep time:
20 minutes

Cook time:
30 minutes

Level:
Moderate

Budget: $$

Omega-3 fats from the salmon, fiber from the asparagus, and carotenoids from the sweet potatoes make this a diabesity-fighting complete meal. Enjoy it any night of the week.

- 1 small sweet potato, peeled and sliced ¼-inch thick
- 1 small yellow onion, sliced ¼-inch thick
- 2 tablespoons extra-virgin olive oil
- sea salt
- 1 garlic clove, minced
- 2 teaspoons dry mustard
- juice and zest of 1 small lemon
- 1 tablespoon chopped fresh rosemary
- 8 ounces asparagus, trimmed
- 2 (4-ounce) skin-on wild salmon fillets

1. Preheat the oven to 425°F.
2. Line a baking sheet with parchment paper. Place the sweet potato and onion slices on the parchment in a single layer. Drizzle with olive oil and sprinkle with salt. Bake for 15 minutes.
3. Meanwhile, mix the garlic, dry mustard, lemon juice, and rosemary to make a paste. Set aside.
4. Remove the baking sheet from the oven, and place the asparagus on the parchment next to the sweet potatoes and onions. Sprinkle the lemon zest on the asparagus. Lay the salmon on top of the asparagus and onions. Spread the mustard paste on top of the salmon.
5. Return the sheet to the oven and roast for 12 minutes. The salmon is done when the flesh flakes with gentle pressure. Serve the salmon on

top of the asparagus, sweet potatoes, and cooked onions. Any left-overs can be refrigerated for up to 3 days.

Nutritional analysis per serving (4 ounces salmon, 1½ cups vegetables): calories 358, fat 18 g, saturated fat 3 g, cholesterol 23 mg, fiber 5 g, protein 34 g, carbohydrate 17 g, sodium 362 mg

Sesame-Crusted Sole with Baby Bok Choy and Wild Rice

Serves: 2

Prep time: 15 minutes

Cook time: 1 hour

Level: Moderate

Budget: $$

Crispy on the outside from the sesame crust yet flaky, moist, and delicate inside, this fish is simple and fast to make. Serving over the crunchy bok choy adds contrast in texture and balance.

WILD RICE:

- ¼ cup uncooked wild rice
- pinch of sea salt
- ¾ cups water

SOLE:

- ¼ cup sesame seeds
- 2 (4-ounce) skinless sole fillets
- 2 tablespoons sesame oil
- 2 heads baby bok choy, trimmed
- 2 garlic cloves, minced
- 1-inch piece fresh ginger, peeled and grated
- sea salt and freshly ground black pepper

MAKE THE WILD RICE:

Put the wild rice, salt, and water in a medium saucepan and bring to a boil. Reduce the heat, cover, and simmer for 50–55 minutes.

MAKE THE SOLE:

1. Place the sesame seeds on a plate. Lightly rub the sole with 1 tablespoon of the sesame oil. Press the sole onto the sesame seeds to form a crust. Set aside.

2. Heat a large skillet over medium-high heat. Add the remaining 1 tablespoon sesame oil and swirl it around the skillet to distribute evenly. Carefully lay the sole in the skillet. Cook the fish until golden brown, approximately 2–3 minutes, leaving it undisturbed to ensure

a crunchy crust. Using a fish spatula, turn the sole over and brown the other side for 2–3 minutes. The fish should flake apart with gentle pressure when done. Remove the sole from the pan and set on a plate.

3. Add the bok choy, garlic, and ginger to the skillet. Toss well, until the bok choy begins to wilt. Season to taste with salt and black pepper. Place the bok choy and steamed wild rice on plates and serve the fish on top. Any leftovers can be refrigerated for up to 4 days.

Nutritional analysis per serving (4 ounces sole, ½ cup rice): calories 469, fat 25 g, saturated fat 3 g, cholesterol 81 mg, fiber 5 g, protein 37 g, carbohydrate 26 g, sodium 265 mg

TOMATO-CRUSTED SOLE WITH GREEN BEANS AND STEAMED WILD RICE

Serves: 2

Prep time:
10 minutes

Cook time:
1 hour

Level:
Moderate

Budget: $$

Plum tomatoes are also called Roma tomatoes. They are available year-round and are versatile and flavorful. Tomatoes are a rich source of the famous carotenoid lycopene, recognized for its cancer-preventive benefits. The extra-virgin olive oil in this recipe ensures that this fat-soluble nutrient will be absorbed better. Think pink when it comes to fruit sources of lycopene.

WILD RICE:

- ¼ cup uncooked wild rice
- pinch of sea salt
- ¾ cups water

SOLE:

- 8 ounces fresh sole, cut into two 4-ounce portions
- 1 shallot, sliced very thinly
- 2 plum tomatoes, sliced into thin circles
- 8 ounces fresh green beans, trimmed
- 2 tablespoons chopped fresh oregano
- sea salt and freshly ground black pepper
- 1 tablespoon extra-virgin olive oil

MAKE THE WILD RICE:

Put the wild rice, salt, and water in a medium saucepan and bring to a boil. Reduce the heat, cover, and simmer for 50–55 minutes.

MAKE THE SOLE:

1. Preheat the oven to 450°F.
2. Place a piece of parchment paper on a baking sheet. Lay the sole pieces on the paper, about 5 inches apart.
3. Place the sliced shallot on top of the sole, followed by the tomatoes. Lay the green beans next to the sole.

4. Sprinkle the fish and green beans with the oregano and salt and black pepper to taste. Drizzle with the olive oil. Bake until the fish flakes apart when tested with a fork, 8–10 minutes.

5. Make a bed of wild rice on a platter and place the fish and green beans on top of the rice. Serve immediately. Any leftovers can be refrigerated for up to 3 days.

Nutritional analysis per serving (4 ounces sole, ¾ cup green beans): calories 363, fat 10 g, saturated fat 0 g, cholesterol 54 mg, fiber 11 g, protein 29 g, carbohydrate 33 g, sodium 213 mg

Tarragon Chicken Salad

Serves: 2

Prep time:
15 minutes

Level: Easy

Budget: $

Watercress is great for detoxification. The cardamom and walnut oil add body and complement the fresh taste of the tarragon. This salad is perfect for those who enjoy a little crunch.

- 8 ounces cooked chicken breast meat, cut into 1-inch pieces
- 3 cups fresh watercress
- 5 radishes, thinly sliced
- 2 celery ribs, thinly sliced
- 1 medium pear, diced
- ⅓ cup pine nuts
- 3 tablespoons chopped fresh tarragon
- ⅛ teaspoon ground cardamom
- 1 tablespoon walnut oil

Combine all of the ingredients in a large salad bowl and toss together until evenly mixed. Serve.

Nutritional analysis per serving (½ cup chicken, 2 cups salad): calories 400, fat 24 g, saturated fat 2 g, cholesterol 68 mg, fiber 5 g, protein 32 g, carbohydrate 18 g, sodium 136 mg

SPICY CHICKEN STIR-FRY

In this gluten-free version of the classic chicken stir-fry, substitute gluten-free tamari for soy sauce. The red chili garlic sauce adds dimension and spice. If you like it hot, add another teaspoon. Serve over hot brown rice if desired.

Serves: 4

Prep time: 20 minutes

Cook time: 15 minutes

Level: Easy

Budget: $

CHICKEN:

- 2 tablespoons low-sodium, gluten-free tamari
- 2 tablespoons rice wine vinegar
- 1 teaspoon sesame oil
- 2 teaspoons arrowroot
- 2 boneless, skinless chicken breasts, sliced

SAUCE:

- ¼ cup low-sodium chicken or vegetable broth
- 1 tablespoon reduced-sodium, gluten-free tamari
- 1 teaspoon rice wine vinegar
- 1 teaspoon sesame oil
- 2 teaspoons chili garlic sauce
- 1 teaspoon arrowroot

STIR-FRY:

- 1 tablespoon peanut oil
- 2 teaspoons red pepper flakes
- 1-inch piece fresh ginger, peeled and grated
- 2 garlic cloves, minced
- 4 scallions, thinly sliced
- 1 (5-ounce) can water chestnuts, drained
- 6 cups baby spinach
- ½ cup roasted peanuts, chopped

MAKE THE CHICKEN:

In a medium bowl whisk together the tamari, rice wine vinegar, sesame oil, and arrowroot. Add the chicken and set aside to marinate for 15–20 minutes.

MAKE THE SAUCE:

In a small bowl whisk together all of the sauce ingredients and set aside.

MAKE THE STIR-FRY:

1. Heat the oil in a wok over high heat. Add the red pepper flakes, ginger, garlic, and scallions and stir-fry, stirring constantly, for 2–3 minutes.
2. Drain the excess marinade from the chicken and add the chicken to the wok. Stir-fry the chicken in the aromatics until mostly cooked through, 1–2 minutes. Pour in the reserved sauce and add the water chestnuts. Finish cooking the chicken in the sauce until it glazes nicely, 3–4 minutes.
3. Reduce the heat to medium and transfer the chicken to a platter, leaving behind as much sauce as possible in the wok.
4. Add the spinach to the wok and stir-fry until it wilts, 3–4 minutes.
5. Serve the chicken with the spinach on the side. Garnish with chopped peanuts. Any leftover stir-fry can be refrigerated for up to 4 days.

Nutritional analysis per serving (1½ cups): calories 215, fat 10 g, saturated fat 1 g, cholesterol 0 mg, fiber 8 g, protein 9 g, carbohydrate 25 g, sodium 155 mg

GINGERED CHICKEN WITH CASHEWS, CARROTS, RAISINS, AND SCALLIONS

Serves: 4

Prep time: 10 minutes

Cook time: 20 minutes

Level: Easy

Budget: $

This one-dish meal couldn't be any easier to make or more satisfying. The ginger adds warmth and is a potent digestive aid. Make sure to garnish with cashews and scallions.

- 1 pound boneless, skinless chicken breasts, sliced
- sea salt and freshly ground black pepper
- 1-inch piece fresh ginger, peeled and grated
- 2 garlic cloves, finely chopped
- 1 tablespoon reduced-sodium, gluten-free tamari
- 3 tablespoons extra-virgin olive oil
- 1 large bunch kale, stemmed and roughly chopped
- 2 large carrots, peeled and chopped
- 6 scallions, finely chopped
- 1 cup roasted cashew halves

1. Season the chicken to taste with salt and black pepper. Mix the chicken, ginger, garlic, and tamari in a medium bowl. Set aside to marinate.

2. Heat 1 tablespoon of the oil in a wok over medium-high heat. After a minute add the kale to the wok and season it to taste with salt. Stir-fry the kale until it is just cooked through, 4–5 minutes. Transfer the kale to a platter.

3. Add the remaining 2 tablespoons oil to the wok and stir-fry the carrots until they soften slightly, 5–6 minutes.

4. Add the chicken and stir-fry until it's firm and cooked through, 3–4 minutes. Turn off the heat and mix in the scallions and cashews. Pour the stir-fried chicken mixture over the kale and serve. Any leftover chicken and greens can be refrigerated for up to 4 days.

Nutritional analysis per serving (4 ounces chicken): calories 277, fat 15 g, saturated fat 3 g, cholesterol 48 mg, fiber 2 g, protein 21 g, carbohydrate 16 g, sodium 132 mg

LEMON ROSEMARY CHICKEN WITH SWISS CHARD AND BAKED DELICATA SQUASH

Serves: 2

Prep time: 15 minutes

Cook time: 25 minutes

Level: Easy

Budget: $

Winter squash, such as delicata, butternut, and acorn, are loaded with colorful carotenoids that are good for the eyes, heart, and lungs. Their sweet, buttery, nutty, creamy flavors make them a delicious addition to many different meals.

- 2 tablespoons extra-virgin olive oil
- 1 delicata squash, halved and seeded
- 1 medium head Swiss chard, stemmed and roughly chopped
- 2 (6-ounce) boneless, skinless chicken breasts
- ¼ cup almond meal
- sea salt and freshly ground black pepper
- ½ cup low-sodium chicken broth
- juice of ½ lemon
- 2 tablespoons chopped fresh rosemary

1. Preheat the oven to 350°F.

2. Brush the cut sides of the squash with 1 teaspoon of the oil. Place the squash, cut sides down, on a baking sheet and roast for 20–25 minutes. The squash is cooked when a knife slides into the flesh easily when pierced. Let the squash cool and remove the skin. Dice the squash into 1-inch cubes and reserve.

3. Heat 1 teaspoon of the oil in a large sauté pan over medium heat. Add the Swiss chard and cook until it wilts, 5–6 minutes. Transfer the greens to a platter.

4. Lay out a 12-inch length of plastic wrap and place the chicken breasts in the center of the plastic wrap. Cover the chicken with a second piece of plastic wrap and pound them with a kitchen mallet until they are about ¼ inch thick.

5. Sprinkle both sides of the chicken breasts with almond meal and salt and black pepper to taste, and set them on a plate.

6. Heat the remaining 4 teaspoons oil in a large sauté pan over medium-high heat. Swirl the oil in the pan to coat the bottom evenly. Carefully add the chicken breasts and cook them for 5 minutes per side.

7. While the chicken cooks, combine the broth, lemon juice, and rosemary in a small bowl and stir until well mixed.

8. When the chicken is golden brown on both sides and cooked through, add the lemon-rosemary mixture to the pan and cook until the sauce reduces and coats the chicken, 2–3 minutes. Serve the chicken on top of the cooked greens with the roasted squash alongside. Any leftover chicken and vegetables can be refrigerated for up to 3 days.

Nutritional analysis per serving (1 chicken breast, 2 cups vegetables): calories 238, fat 10 g, saturated fat 2 g, cholesterol 60 mg, fiber 8 g, protein 26 g, carbohydrate 15 g, sodium 479 mg

Moroccan Chicken with Cauliflower and Cashews

Serves: 4

Prep time:
30 Minutes

Cook time:
30 minutes

Level: Easy

Budget: $

The garam masala adds a satisfying intensity to the flavors infusing the chicken. The chickpeas and cauliflower soak up the spices and turn a beautiful, rich color.

- 1 tablespoon extra-virgin olive oil
- 1 pound boneless, skinless chicken breasts, cut into 1-inch cubes
- 1 small onion, chopped
- 3 garlic cloves, minced
- 2 cups cauliflower florets
- 2 cups cooked chickpeas or 1 (15-ounce) can chickpeas, rinsed and drained
- 6 cups low-sodium chicken broth
- 2 tablespoons pomegranate molasses
- 1 tablespoon garam masala
- ½ cup raw cashews, chopped, for garnish

1. Preheat the oven to 350°F.
2. Heat the oil in a large Dutch oven over medium-high heat. Add the chicken pieces and cook them, stirring occasionally, until brown, 3–4 minutes.
3. Add the onion, garlic, cauliflower, chickpeas, broth, pomegranate molasses, and garam masala, and stir until well mixed.
4. Cover the pot and place it on the bottom rack of the oven. Cook until the vegetables are tender and the chicken is cooked through, about 25 minutes.
5. Transfer the chicken and vegetables to a serving dish and garnish with the chopped cashews. Any leftover chicken and vegetables can be refrigerated for up to 3 days.

Nutritional analysis per serving (1¼ cups): calories 515, fat 17 g, saturated fat 1 g, cholesterol 17 mg, fiber 7 g, protein 45 g, carbohydrate 47 g, sodium 960 mg

Lime-Scented Turkey with Sautéed Vegetables and Steamed Brown Rice

Serves: 4

Prep time: 20 minutes

Cook time: 45 minutes

Level: Easy

Budget: $

The lime in this dish is incredibly fragrant and fresh. D–limonene is found in lime zest and is known to inhibit cancer and boost immunity.

RICE:

- 2 cups water
- ½ teaspoon sea salt
- 1 cup uncooked brown rice

TURKEY:

- zest and juice of 1 lime
- 1 cup low-sodium chicken broth
- 2 teaspoons arrowroot
- ½ teaspoon garam masala
- 1 tablespoon extra-virgin olive oil
- 1 pound turkey tenderloins
- sea salt and freshly ground black pepper
- 1 medium red bell pepper, seeded and sliced
- 1 baby eggplant, sliced
- 2 medium yellow onions, sliced
- 4 large carrots, peeled and sliced on the diagonal
- 2 garlic cloves, minced

MAKE THE RICE:

Heat the water in a small saucepan over high heat. When it boils, add the rice and reduce the heat to low. Cover the pot and simmer until all the liquid has evaporated and the rice is tender, 35–45 minutes. Turn off the heat and allow the rice to steam for 3 minutes with the lid on. Fluff the rice and set aside.

MAKE THE TURKEY:

1. In a small bowl, whisk together the lime juice and zest, broth, arrowroot, and garam masala until evenly mixed. Set aside.

2. Heat the oil in a large cast-iron pan over medium-high heat. Add the turkey to the pan and season to taste with salt and black pepper. Cook, turning occasionally, until brown, about 5 minutes.

3. Add the bell pepper, eggplant, onions, carrots, and garlic, and cook until the vegetables are tender but still crisp, 4–5 minutes.

4. Pour in the sauce and toss the turkey and vegetables until they are evenly coated in the sauce. Remove from the heat.

5. Spread out the rice on a platter to form a bed. Spoon the turkey and vegetables over the rice. Any leftover turkey and vegetables can be stored in the refrigerator for up to 3 days.

Nutritional analysis per serving (4 ounces turkey, 1½ cups vegetables, ½ cup rice): calories 359, fat 6 g, saturated fat 1 g, cholesterol 71 mg, fiber 5 g, protein 32 g, carbohydrate 43 g, sodium 194 mg

OVEN ROASTED TURKEY BURGERS WITH BRUSSELS SPROUTS AND BAKED SWEET POTATOES

Serves: 4

Prep time: 10 minutes

Cook time: 30 minutes

Level: Easy

Budget: $

The addition of button mushrooms and fresh sage boosts the antioxidant value of these delicious burgers.

VEGETABLES:

- 1 pound Brussels sprouts, trimmed
- 2 medium sweet potatoes, peeled and cut into ¼-inch thick wedges
- 1 teaspoon extra-virgin olive oil
- sea salt and freshly ground black pepper

BURGERS:

- 1 pound lean ground turkey
- 4 ounces white button mushrooms, chopped
- ½ small yellow onion, minced
- 1 celery rib, minced
- 2 tablespoons finely chopped fresh parsley
- 1 tablespoon reduced-sodium, gluten-free tamari
- 1 tablespoon chopped fresh sage
- 1 garlic clove, finely chopped
- 1 teaspoon extra-virgin olive oil

MAKE THE VEGETABLES:

1. Preheat the oven to 400°F.
2. Place the Brussels sprouts and sweet potato wedges in a roasting pan and drizzle them with the oil. Season the vegetables to taste with salt and black pepper, and place them in the oven for 30 minutes until lightly browned.

MAKE THE BURGERS:

1. While the vegetables are roasting, in a medium bowl combine all of the burger ingredients except for the oil. Mix everything together until the vegetables are evenly distributed throughout the meat.

145

2. Form the mixture into four equal patties. Grease a baking sheet with the oil and place the patties on the baking sheet.

3. Roast the turkey burgers for 15 minutes, flipping them once halfway through the cooking. (You can also grill the burgers for approximately 7–8 minutes on each side.)

4. Serve the burgers with the roasted vegetables on the side. Leftover uncooked patties and vegetables can be stored in the refrigerator for up to 2 days.

Nutritional analysis per serving (1 burger, 1 cup vegetables): calories 494, fat 21 g, saturated fat 3 g, cholesterol 84 mg, fiber 7 g, protein 27 g, carbohydrate 34 g, sodium 231 mg

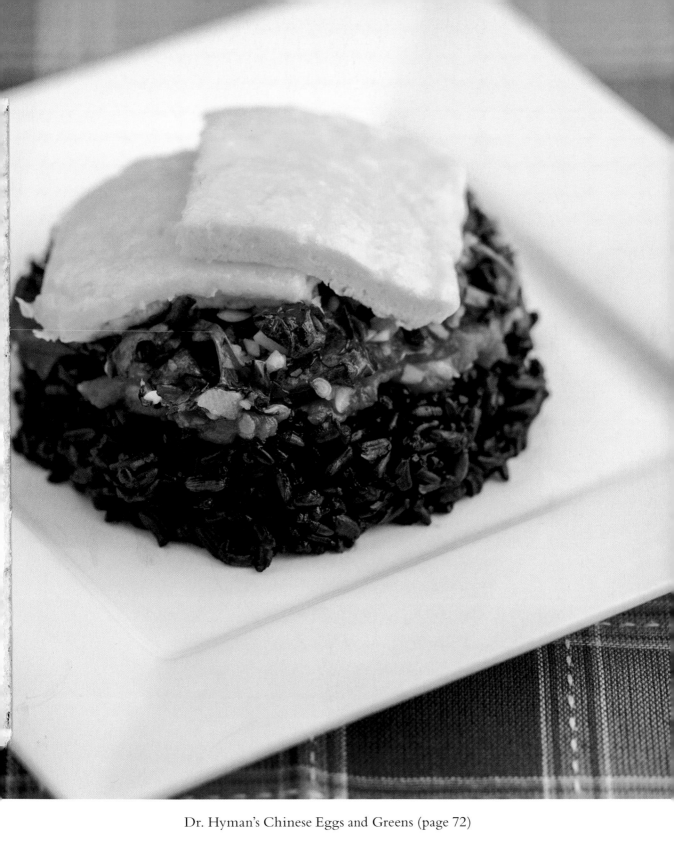

Dr. Hyman's Chinese Eggs and Greens (page 72)

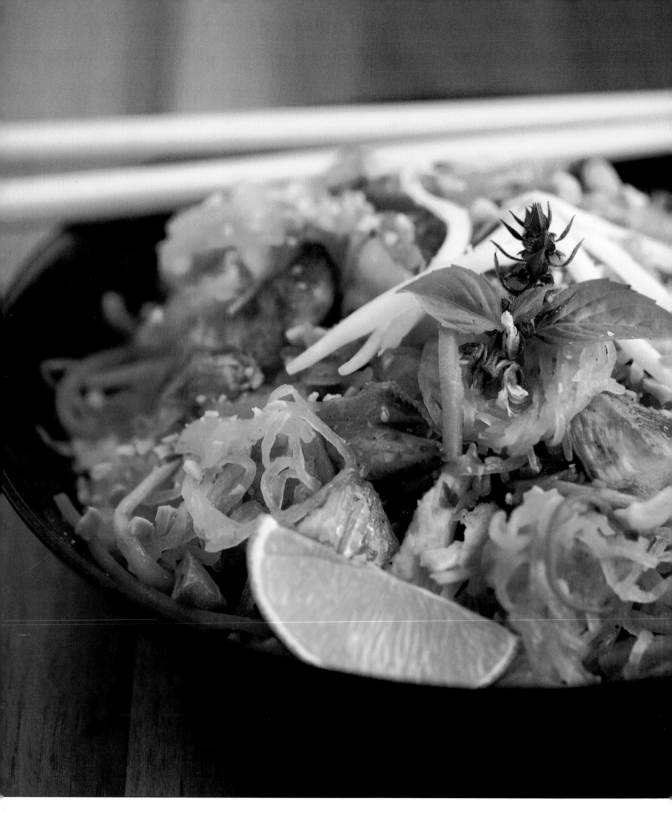

Spaghetti Squash Pad Thai (page 119)

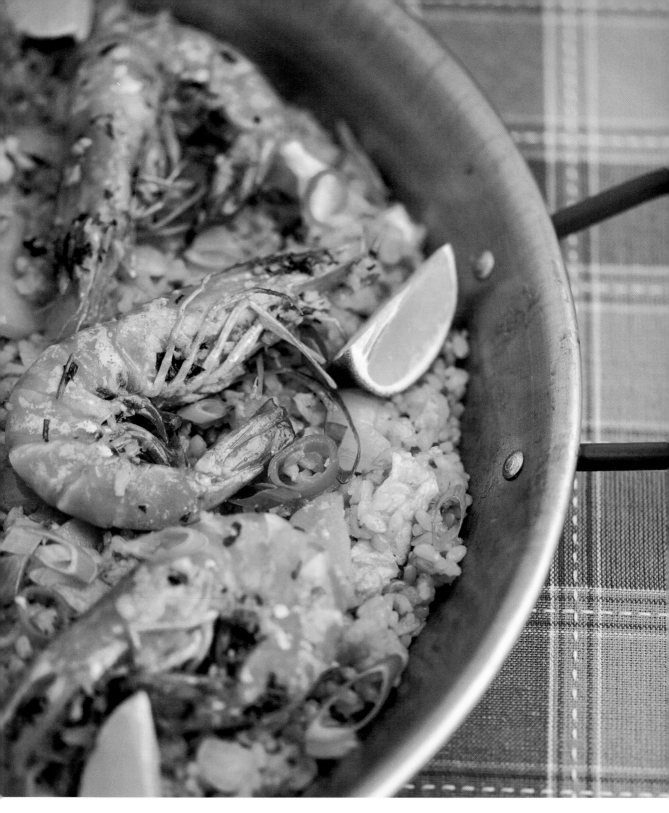

Asian Prawn Paella (page 123)

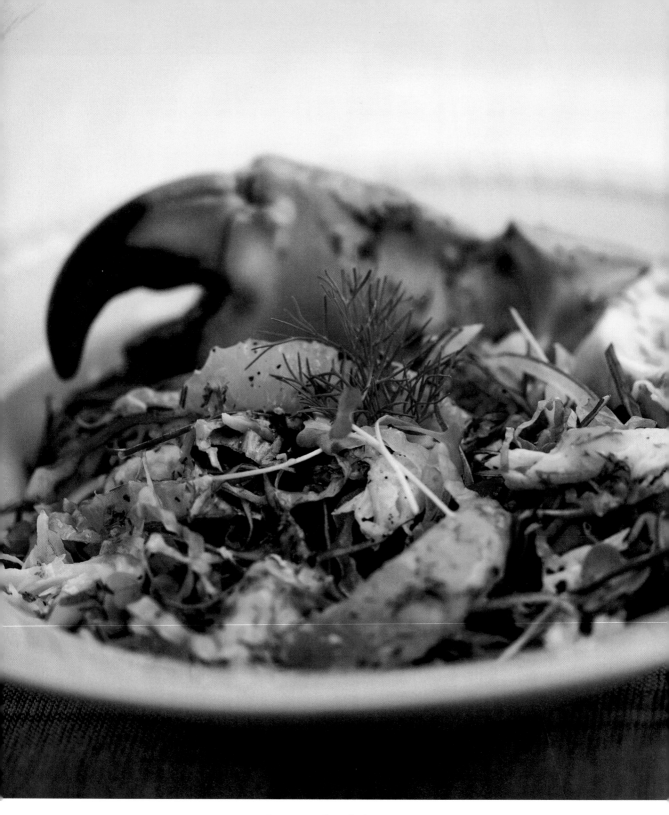

Citrus Crab Salad (page 125)

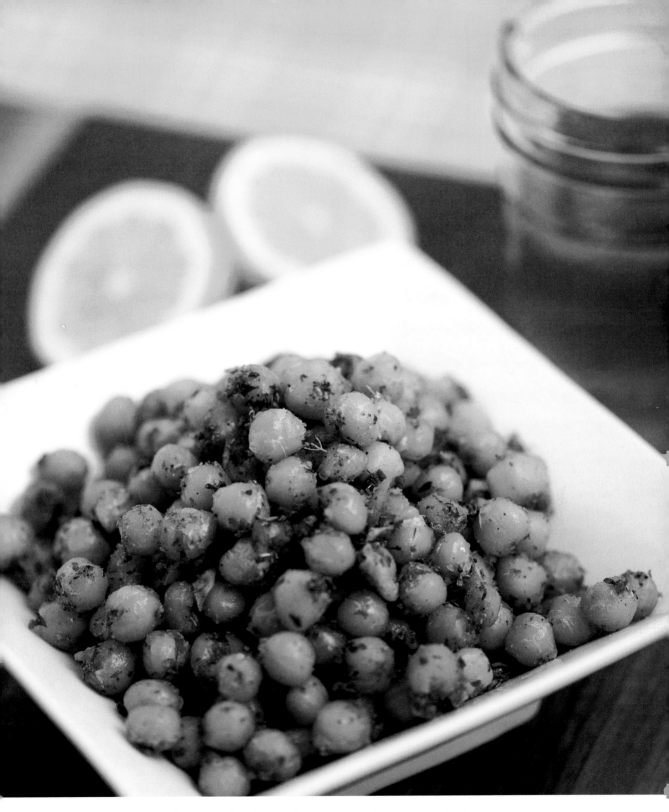

Lemony Greek Pan–Roasted Chickpeas (page 153)

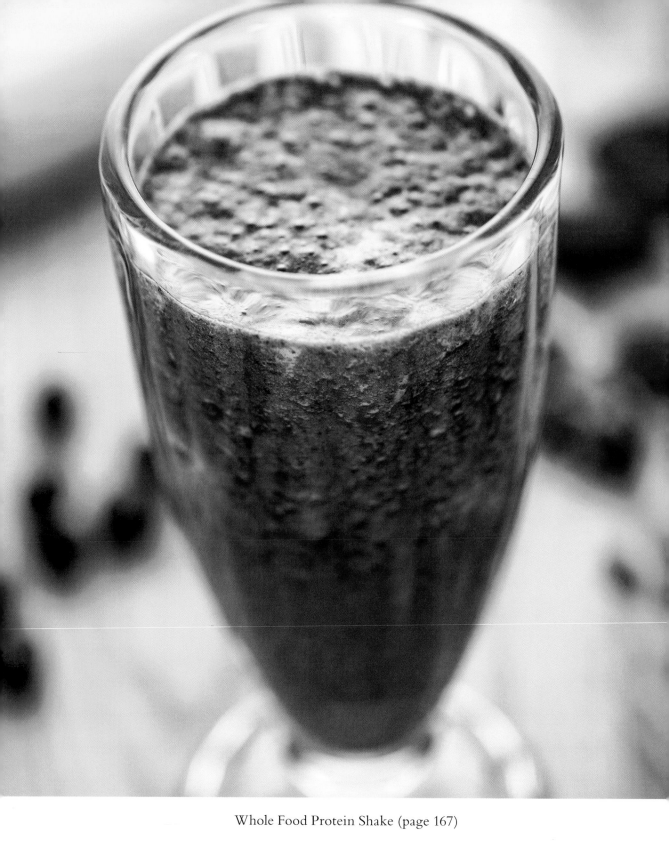

Whole Food Protein Shake (page 167)

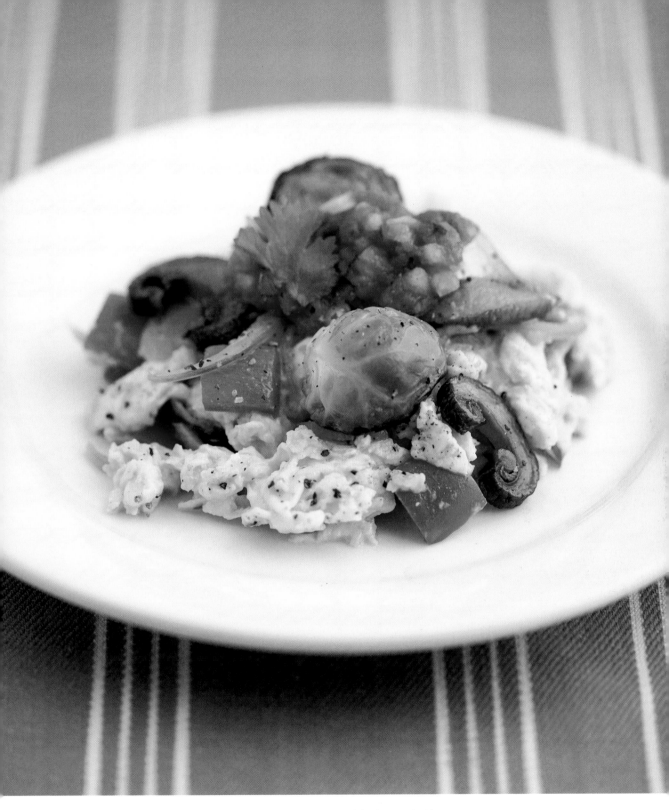

Weekday Veggie Scramble (page 173)

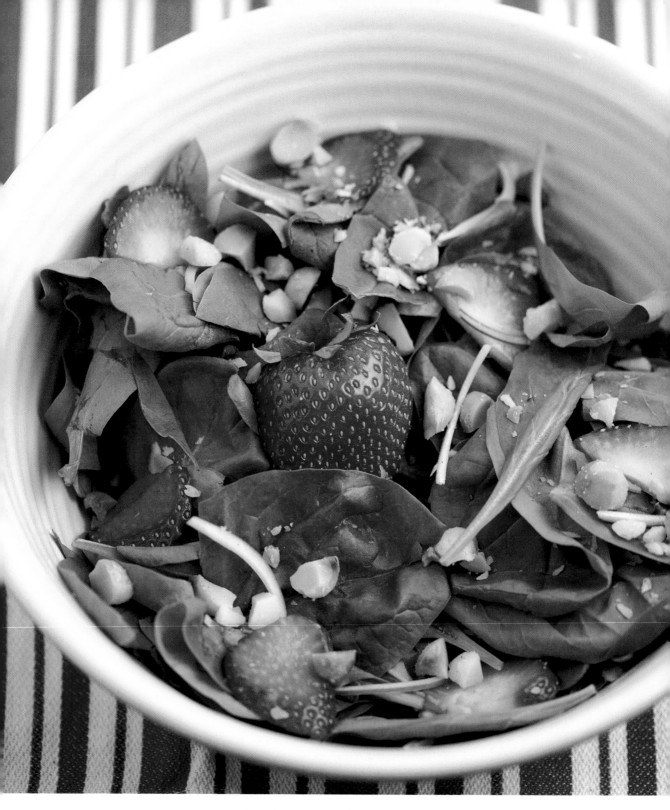

Strawberry Spinach Salad (page 195)

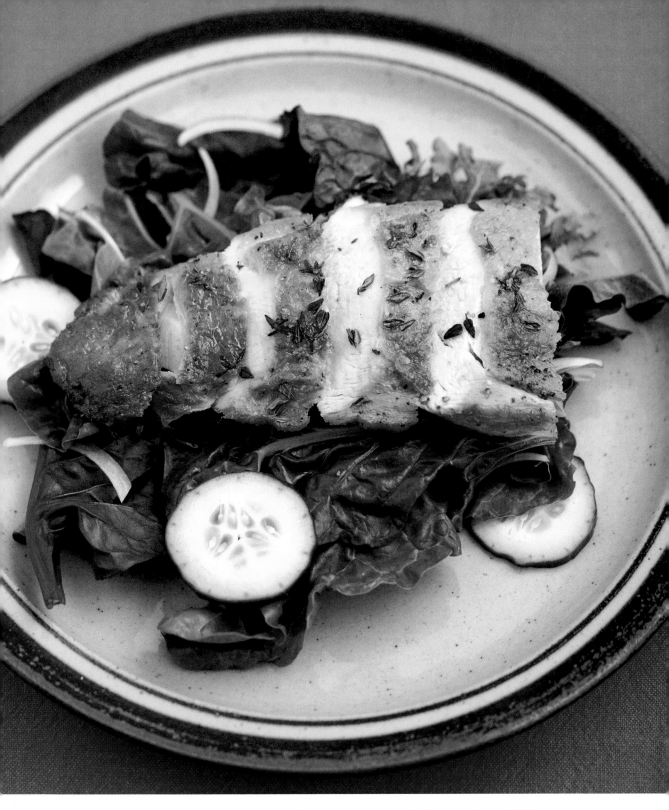

Roast Turkey Breast and Avocado Cream on a Bed of Greens (page 230)

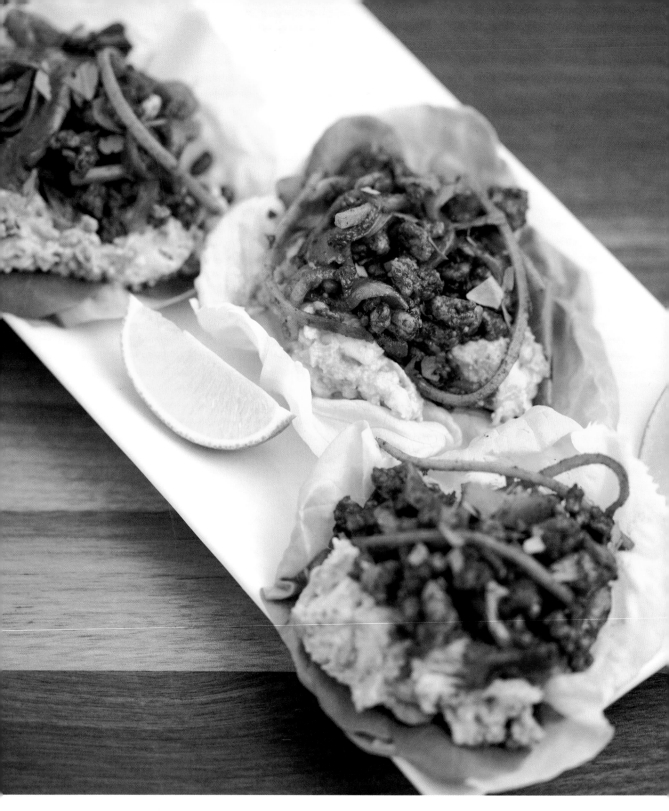

Spiced Ground Turkey Wrap with Watercress and Avocado (page 232)

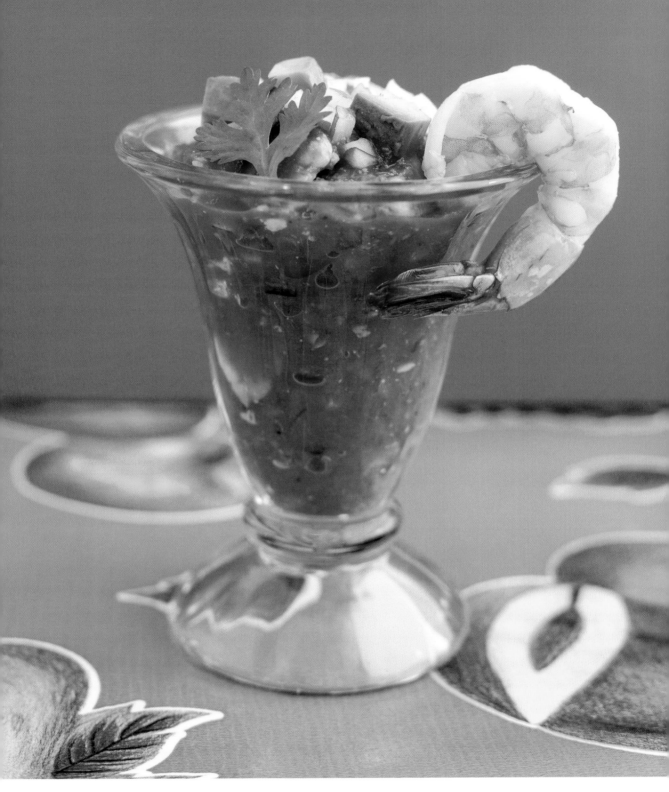

Shrimp Salsa (page 251)

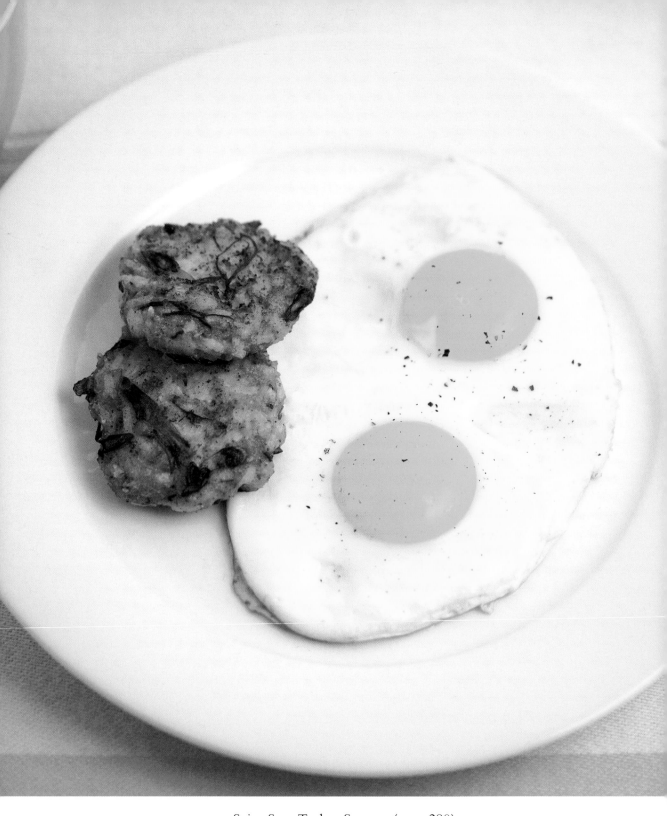

Spicy Sage Turkey Sausage (page 280)

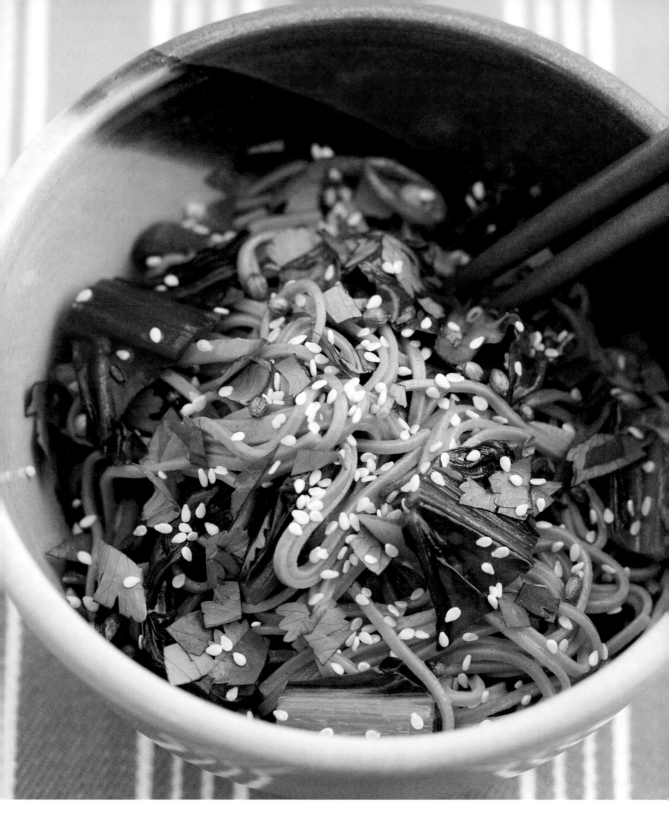

Hearty Greens with Ginger and Sugar Snap Peas over Soba (page 296)

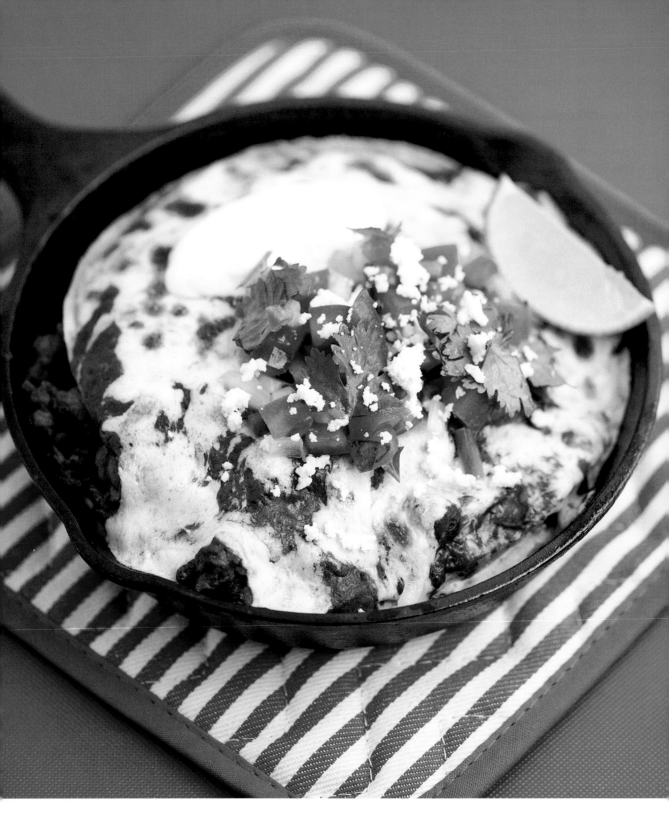

Mexican Lasagna (page 309)

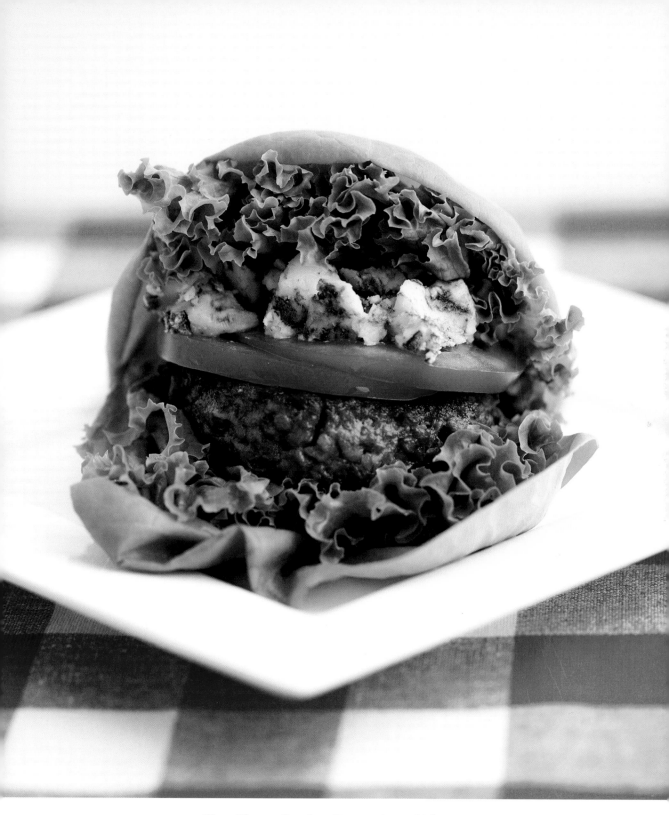

Blue Cheese Cowboy Burger (page 311)

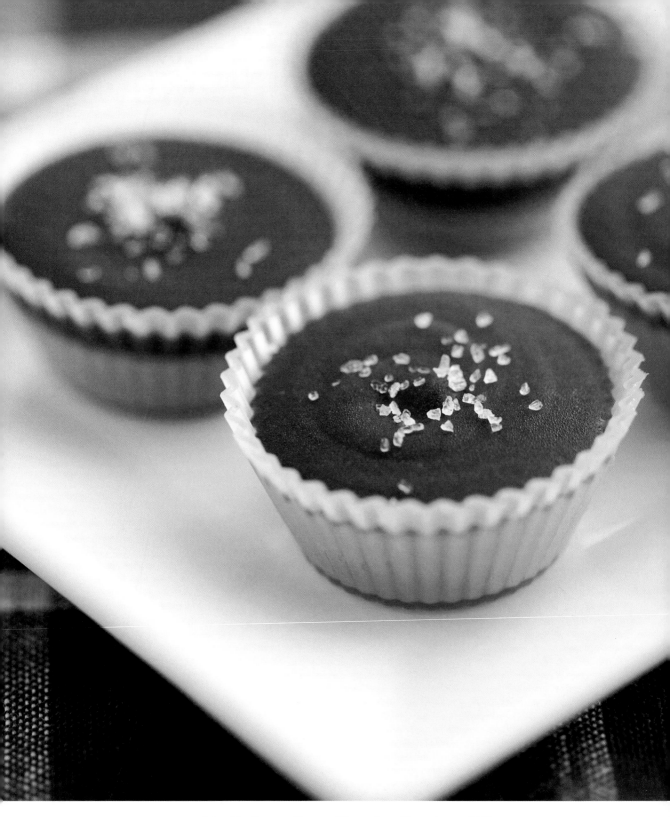

Double Peanut Butter Chocolate Cups (page 325)

BEEF AND CABBAGE CASSEROLE

For those nights when a simple yet deeply satisfying meal is desired, choose this casserole for your friends and family. Use grass-fed beef to increase your omega-3 fat intake. Make your own salsa or buy it fresh.

Serves: 8

Prep time: 20 minutes

Cook time: 1 hour 30 minutes

Level: Easy

Budget: $$

STEW:

- 1 tablespoon extra-virgin olive oil
- 1 pound lean ground beef
- sea salt and freshly ground black pepper
- 1 medium yellow onion, chopped
- 1 large carrot, peeled and shredded
- 1 medium head green cabbage, roughly chopped
- 2 cups low-sodium beef broth
- 1 cup uncooked long-grain brown rice

SALSA:

- 2 medium plum tomatoes, finely chopped
- ½ small white onion, chopped
- 1 garlic clove, minced
- 1 small jalapeño pepper, seeded and finely chopped
- ¼ cup chopped fresh cilantro
- juice of 2 limes

MAKE THE STEW:

1. Preheat the oven to 350°F.
2. Heat the oil in a medium oven-safe pot over medium-high heat. Add the beef, season to taste with salt and black pepper, and break it up as it cooks. Once most of the beef has browned, after 8–10 minutes, add the onions and cook them in the beef juices until soft.
3. Toss the carrots and cabbage into the pan and pour in the broth. When it boils, add the rice, turn off the heat, and cover the pot with a tight-fitting lid.
4. Put the pot in the oven and bake for 1 hour.

MAKE THE SALSA:

Combine all of the ingredient for the salsa in a small bowl and mix well. Season to taste with salt and let it sit for 30–40 minutes while the casserole finishes cooking.

ASSEMBLE THE STEW:

Remove the pot from the oven and pour the casserole into a serving dish. Serve garnished with a tablespoon or two of the fresh salsa on each portion. Leftovers can be stored in the refrigerator for up to 4 days.

Nutritional analysis per serving (1⅓ cups): calories 232, fat 6 g, saturated fat 2 g, cholesterol 38 mg, fiber 4 g, protein 16 g, carbohydrate 28 g, sodium 366 mg

Teriyaki Beef Vegetable Kabobs

Serves: 4

Prep time: 3 hours 20 minutes

Cook time: 15 minutes

Level: Easy

Budget: $

Teriyaki is a favorite for kids and adults alike. This tasty dish will go a long way toward pleasing the whole family and keeping you fit and healthy at the same time. But remember, you don't want to eat red meat too often.

TERIYAKI MARINADE:

- ¼ cup reduced-sodium, gluten-free tamari
- 2 tablespoons rice vinegar
- 1 tablespoon Dijon mustard
- 2 teaspoons toasted sesame oil
- 1 teaspoon grated fresh ginger
- 1 garlic clove, minced

KABOBS:

- 1 pound sirloin, trimmed and cut into 1-inch cubes
- 1 large red onion, cut into 1-inch wedges
- 1 zucchini, cut into 1-inch chunks
- 1 yellow bell pepper, seeded and cut into 1-inch chunks
- 1 orange bell pepper, seeded and cut into 1-inch chunks
- 8 cherry tomatoes
- 8 cremini mushrooms, stemmed
- 2 medium sweet potatoes, peeled and cut into ¼-inch slices
- 1 tablespoon extra-virgin olive oil

MAKE THE TERIYAKI MARINADE:

Whisk together all of the marinade ingredients in a small bowl until blended.

KABOBS:

1. Place the vegetables and beef onto eight metal skewers, alternating between the meat and vegetables as you stack them. Place the kabobs in a shallow baking dish and brush them liberally with the teriyaki marinade. Marinate in the refrigerator for at least 2 hours.

2. Preheat the grill. When hot, brush the grill grates with oil.

3. Put the kabobs on the grill and pour over any remaining marinade. Cook, turning the kabobs once halfway through the cooking, until cooked to your desired degree of doneness (about 6 minutes total for medium-rare, or 8 minutes for medium.)

4. When cooked, transfer the kabobs to a platter and let them rest for 3–4 minutes before serving. Uncooked kabobs can be stored in the marinade for up to 24 hours in the refrigerator.

Nutritional analysis per serving (2 kabobs): calories 323, fat 14 g, saturated fat 5 g, cholesterol 76 mg, fiber 3 g, protein 27 g, carbohydrate 21 g, sodium 708 mg

BEEF AND BEAN TACOS

To really make this a winner for the Blood Sugar Solution, use grass-fed sirloin. Garnish with avocado and fresh salsa.

- 2 tablespoons grapeseed oil
- 1 medium yellow onion, chopped
- 4 garlic cloves, minced
- 2 teaspoons chili powder
- 2 teaspoons ground cumin
- 1 teaspoon dried oregano
- 1 pound lean ground beef
- sea salt and freshly ground black pepper
- 2 cups cooked pinto beans or 1 (15-ounce) can pinto beans, drained, liquid reserved
- 1 tablespoon hot pepper sauce
- juice of 1 lime
- 6–8 soft sprouted corn tortillas
- ¼ cup cilantro leaves, for garnish
- 1 lime, cut into wedges, for garnish

1. Heat the oil in a large cast-iron pan over medium-high heat. Once hot, add the onion, garlic, chili powder, cumin, and oregano and cook, stirring frequently, until the onions are soft and starting to caramelize, 6–8 minutes.

2. Add the beef and season to taste with salt and black pepper. Cook the beef in the spices, breaking it up as it cooks, until brown, 8–10 minutes.

3. Pour in the beans along with the reserved bean liquid or 1 cup of water if using cooked beans. Use a wooden spoon to lift any browned bits of beef that might be stuck to the bottom of the pan, and stir them into the beans and beef.

4. Add the hot sauce and lime juice and mix well. Transfer the taco meat to a bowl.

Serves: 4

Prep time: 15 minutes

Cook time: 20 minutes

Level: Easy

Budget: $

5. Warm the tortillas on a dry griddle or skillet and fill them with the taco meat. Garnish with a few leaves of cilantro and lime wedges, and serve immediately. Any leftover filling can be refrigerated for up to 3 days.

Nutritional analysis per serving (1 taco): calories 341, fat 11 g, saturated fat 5 g, cholesterol 75 mg, fiber 15 g, protein 32 g, carbohydrate 37 g, sodium 531 mg

SNACKS AND SIDES

LEMONY GREEK PAN-ROASTED CHICKPEAS

Serves: 4

Prep time: 5 minutes

Cook time: 1 hour 20 minutes

Level: Easy

Budget: $

Oregano, parsley, and garlic give your body an anti-inflammatory boost while stimulating your senses. Serve these chickpeas along with your main dish or enjoy them alone as a nutrient-dense snack.

INFUSED LEMON OIL:

- ¼ cup grapeseed oil
- zest of ½ large lemon

CHICKPEAS:

- 2 cups cooked chickpeas or 1 (15-ounce) can chickpeas, rinsed and drained
- 2 teaspoons dried oregano
- 2 teaspoons dried parsley
- 2 teaspoons garlic powder
- sea salt and freshly ground black pepper

MAKE THE INFUSED OIL:

Combine the oil and lemon zest in a small pot over medium heat. Heat until the oil is warm, about 1 minute. Turn off the heat, and let the pot sit for 1 hour.

MAKE THE CHICKPEAS:

1. In a medium bowl mix the chickpeas with the herbs until they are fully coated.
2. Heat the lemon oil in a medium cast-iron pan over medium-high heat. Once the oil is hot add the chickpeas to the pan.
3. Reduce the heat to medium-low and season the chickpeas to taste with salt and black pepper. Cook, stirring, until the chickpeas are brown and slightly crispy on the edges, about 15 minutes. Transfer to

a plate, let cool briefly, and serve. Any leftovers can be refrigerated for up to 4 days.

Nutritional analysis per serving (½ cup): calories 80, fat 1 g, saturated fat 0 g, cholesterol 0 mg, fiber 3 g, protein 4 g, carbohydrate 12 g, sodium 133 mg (based on ⅛ teaspoon sea salt)

GINGER EDAMAME SALAD

Savory snacks are a real treat, especially when they are as simple to prepare as this one. The tamari and ginger transform everyday edamame into a unique snack that will satisfy both your taste buds and your blood sugar.

- 2 teaspoons grapeseed oil
- 1-inch piece fresh ginger, peeled and grated
- 2 cups frozen edamame, in shell
- 2 tablespoons reduced-sodium, gluten-free tamari
- 1 teaspoon pure maple syrup

| Serves: 4 |
| Prep time: 5 minutes |
| Cook time: 8 minutes |
| Level: Easy |
| Budget: $ |

1. Heat the oil in a wok over medium-high heat. Once hot, add the ginger and stir-fry until aromatic, about 30 seconds.

2. Pour in the edamame and constantly toss them in the ginger for 2–3 minutes.

3. Add the tamari and maple syrup and toss until the edamame are nicely glazed in the sauce. Serve immediately. Any leftovers can be refrigerated for up to 4 days.

Nutritional analysis per serving (⅓ cup): calories 122, fat 5 g, saturated fat 0 g, cholesterol 0 mg, fiber 4 g, protein 9 g, carbohydrate 9 g, sodium 318 mg

TASTY BLACK RICE

Serves: 6

Prep time:
5 minutes

Cook time:
40 minutes

Level: Easy

Budget: $

This simple recipe adds variety and spice to a basic side dish. It can also be cooked in a rice cooker for convenience.

- 1 cup uncooked black rice
- 2 cups water
- 2 teaspoons extra-virgin olive oil
- ½ teaspoon sea salt
- ½ teaspoon chopped fresh thyme
- ¼ teaspoon onion powder
- 1 bay leaf

1. Combine all of the ingredients in a small pot, cover, and bring to a boil over high heat. Reduce the heat to low and simmer, covered, until all of the liquid has evaporated and the rice is tender, 30–35 minutes.

2. Remove the pot from the heat and let the rice steam with the lid on for 5 minutes.

3. Remove the bay leaf from the rice and serve hot. Leftover rice can be refrigerated for up to 5 days.

Nutritional analysis per serving (⅓ cup): calories 193, fat 4 g, saturated fat 1 g, cholesterol 0 mg, fiber 2 g, protein 4 g, carbohydrate 36 g, sodium 132 mg

SPICY BROWN RICE

This simple recipe adds variety and spice to this staple in our side dish category. It can also be cooked in a rice cooker for convenience.

- 1 cup uncooked short-grain brown rice
- 2 cups water
- 1 garlic clove, minced
- ¼ teaspoon ground turmeric
- ¼ teaspoon cayenne pepper
- ½ teaspoon sea salt

Serves: 6

Prep time: 5 minutes

Cook time: 30 minutes

Level: Easy

Budget: $

1. Combine all of the ingredients in a small pot, cover, and bring to a boil over high heat. Reduce the heat to low and simmer, covered, until all of the liquid has evaporated and the rice is tender, 25–30 minutes.

2. Remove the pot from the heat and let the rice steam with the lid on for 3–4 minutes, then serve. Leftover rice can be refrigerated for up to 5 days.

Nutritional analysis per serving (⅓ cup): calories 173, fat 1 g, saturated fat 0 g, cholesterol 0 mg, fiber 2 g, protein 4 g, carbohydrate 36 g, sodium 132 mg

Quinoa and Avocado Salad

Serves: 3

Prep time:
10 minutes

Cook time:
30 minutes

Level: Easy

Budget: $

Adding nuts to any salad is a great way to increase protein value and fiber. Combining a little bit of olive oil with kale, avocado, onions, lemon, and pepper mixed with quinoa adds good-quality fats, protein, and antioxidants to your lunch.

QUINOA:

- 1 cup uncooked quinoa
- 1½ cup water
- ½ teaspoon sea salt

SALAD:

- 1 large bunch kale, stemmed and chopped
- 1 avocado, peeled, pitted, and chopped
- ¾ cup walnuts, chopped
- ½ medium red onion, chopped
- juice of 1 large lemon
- 2 tablespoons extra-virgin olive oil
- sea salt and freshly ground black pepper

MAKE THE QUINOA:

1. Dry-toast the quinoa in a medium pot over medium-high heat until aromatic, 3–4 minutes.

2. Add the water and salt and bring to a boil. Cover the pan, reduce the heat to low, and simmer until all of the liquid has evaporated and the quinoa is cooked, about 25 minutes. Turn off the heat and let the quinoa steam in the pot for 3–5 minutes with the lid on.

3. Fluff the quinoa with a fork and transfer to a large bowl.

ASSEMBLE THE SALAD:

Add the kale, avocado, nuts, and onion to the bowl of quinoa. Add the lemon juice to the quinoa and pour over the oil. Season to taste with salt and black pepper and lightly toss the salad to coat everything evenly. Serve chilled or at room temperature. Store any leftovers in the refrigerator for up to 5 days.

Nutritional analysis per serving (1 cup): calories 474, fat 28 g, saturated fat 3 g, cholesterol 0 mg, fiber 12 g, protein 14 g, carbohydrate 47 g, sodium 349 mg

ASIAN QUINOA SALAD

Serves: 8

Prep time: 10 minutes

Cook time: 30 minutes

Level: Easy

Budget: $

The black and white sesame seeds, cilantro, cabbage, quinoa, and spinach make a refreshing and unique salad. Tamari provides a good source of fiber and protein in the delicious dressing

QUINOA:

- 2 cups uncooked quinoa
- 3 cups low-sodium chicken broth
- ½ small head red cabbage, finely sliced
- 2 celery ribs, finely sliced
- 4 shallots, finely sliced
- 1 cup chopped fresh cilantro
- 2 tablespoons white sesame seeds
- 2 tablespoons black sesame seeds
- 8 ounces baby spinach

DRESSING:

- 2 garlic cloves, peeled
- ⅓ cup reduced-sodium, gluten-free tamari
- 1 tablespoon rice vinegar
- 1-inch piece fresh ginger, peeled and grated
- freshly ground black pepper to taste
- ⅓ cup extra-virgin olive oil

MAKE THE QUINOA:

1. Dry-toast the quinoa in a medium pot over medium-high heat until aromatic, 3–4 minutes.
2. Add the broth and bring to a boil. Cover the pan, reduce the heat to low, and simmer until all of the liquid has evaporated, about 25 minutes. Turn off the heat and let the quinoa steam in the pot for 3–5 minutes with the lid on.

3. Fluff the quinoa with a fork and, while hot, add the cabbage, celery, shallots, and cilantro. Put the lid back on and let the vegetables steam for a couple of minutes over the quinoa.

4. Heat a small pan over medium heat and dry-toast the sesame seeds until golden brown, 3–4 minutes. Add the toasted seeds to the quinoa and vegetable mixture and gently fold to combine.

5. Transfer the quinoa and vegetables to a large bowl and stir in the spinach.

MAKE THE DRESSING:

Combine all of the dressing ingredients except the oil in a blender. Blend on medium speed while slowly pouring in the oil. Blend until smooth. Taste for seasoning and add more black pepper if desired.

ASSEMBLE THE SALAD:

Pour the dressing over the quinoa and vegetables and gently toss until coated evenly. Serve. Any leftovers can be stored in the refrigerator for up to 4 days.

Nutritional analysis per serving (1 cup): calories 275, fat 13 g, saturated fat 2 g, cholesterol 0 mg, fiber 5 g, protein 9 g, carbohydrate 32 g, sodium 217 mg

Quinoa with Citrus Vinaigrette

Serves: 10

Prep time: 10 minutes

Cook time: 30 minutes

Level: Easy

Budget: $

This dish is a delightful combination of veggies, and the orange zest infuses a tangy flavor into the salad. It makes a wonderful side dish to any meal.

QUINOA:

- 1 cup uncooked quinoa
- 1½ cup water
- ½ teaspoon sea salt

CITRUS VINAIGRETTE:

- juice of 1 lime
- juice of 1 small lemon
- zest of 1 orange
- 2 garlic cloves, minced
- ½ small Vidalia onion, chopped
- 4 fresh basil leaves
- 2 tablespoons chopped fresh parsley
- ¼ cup extra-virgin olive oil
- sea salt and freshly ground black pepper

SALAD:

- 1 large red bell pepper, seeded and chopped
- 1 cup fresh or thawed frozen corn
- 1 small cucumber, chopped
- 1 medium tomato, chopped

MAKE THE QUINOA:

1. Dry-toast the quinoa in a medium pot over medium-high heat until aromatic, 3–4 minutes.

2. Add the water and salt and bring to a boil. Cover the pan, reduce the heat to low, and simmer until all of the liquid has evaporated and the

quinoa is cooked, about 25 minutes. Turn off the heat and let the quinoa steam in the pot for 3–5 minutes with the lid on.

3. Fluff the quinoa with a fork and transfer to a large bowl.

MAKE THE CITRUS VINAIGRETTE:

Combine the citrus juices and zest, garlic, onion, basil, and parsley in a blender. Blend on medium speed while slowly pouring in the oil. Season to taste with salt and black pepper and blend until well mixed, about 2 minutes.

ASSEMBLE THE SALAD:

Add the bell pepper, corn, cucumber, and tomato to the bowl of quinoa. Drizzle the dressing over the quinoa and lightly toss it to coat everything evenly. Serve chilled or at room temperature. Store any leftovers in the refrigerator for up to 5 days.

Nutritional analysis per serving (½ cup): calories 154, fat 8 g, saturated fat 1 g, cholesterol 0 mg, fiber 3 g, protein 4 g, carbohydrate 21 g, sodium 70 mg

ROASTED VEGGIES TO MAKE YOUR LIVER HAPPY

Serves: 4

Prep time:
10 minutes

Cook time:
30 minutes

Level: Easy

Budget: $

Not only do the colors make this dish a pleasurable addition to your dinner, but the warmth and hearty texture from the roasted vegetables are perfect for those chilly fall and winter nights. The beets, onion, and garlic are especially great for boosting your detoxification.

- 1 large sweet potato, peeled and cut into 2-inch chunks
- 2 large beets, cut into 2-inch chunks
- 2 large yellow onions, quartered
- 4 garlic cloves, peeled
- 2 tablespoons extra-virgin coconut oil
- sea salt and freshly ground black pepper
- 1 teaspoon extra-virgin olive oil

1. Preheat the oven to 350°F.
2. Combine all of the vegetables in a large bowl and toss them in the coconut oil. Spread the vegetables out in an even layer in a roasting pan and season them generously with salt and black pepper. Roast, stirring occasionally to prevent burning, until the vegetables are brown and soft, 20–30 minutes. Let cool for 5 minutes, drizzle with the olive oil, and serve. Any leftovers can be refrigerated for up to 4 days.

Nutritional analysis per serving (½ cup): calories 131, fat 24 g, saturated fat 6 g, cholesterol 0 mg, fiber 3 g, protein 2 g, carbohydrate 17 g, sodium 342 mg

5

The Advanced Plan

INTRODUCTION

The Advanced Plan is designed for those with more advanced diabesity and everyone with full-blown type 2 diabetes. The quiz on page 10 will help you determine if you have advanced diabesity. This plan will shut down sugar and insulin spikes and begin the process of rebooting your metabolism. If you have had trouble losing weight or struggled with carb or sugar cravings, the Advanced Plan will quickly shut them down and help you lose weight faster. Not in weeks or months but in hours to days. Over time your cells will work better, you will produce less insulin, and your body will become more resilient. Anyone can start with the Advanced Plan even if you don't have advanced diabesity—the results will be more dramatic.

The Advanced Plan starts with all the guidelines from the Basic Plan—whole, fresh, real food including nuts, seeds, fruits, vegetables, whole grains, beans, lean animal protein, and high-quality fats. The Basic Plan also starts with unjunking your diet from processed foods, flours and sugars, and eliminating the most common inflammatory foods, including gluten and dairy. The Advanced Plan goes one step further—it eliminates all grains and starchy vegetables (sweet potatoes and winter squash) and limits fruit to ½ cup of berries a day. Beans should be kept to a minimum (no more than ½ cup a day). These added changes will reduce the glycemic load, or sugar-spiking quality of your diet, even further, allowing your body to heal from diabesity. Now enjoy all these wonderful recipes that illustrate the delightful flavors and abundance in a healing diet using food as medicine. Remember, your grocery store should be your pharmacy.

BREAKFAST

WHOLE FOOD PROTEIN SHAKE

Serves: 3

Prep time:
5 minutes

Level: Easy

Budget: $$

This shake will power you through the hardest and longest of days. It is 100% whole, fresh, real food, with a spotlight on healthy fats and potent antioxidants from the blueberries.

- 1 cup frozen blueberries
- 2 tablespoons almond butter
- 2 tablespoons pumpkin seeds
- 2 tablespoons chia seeds
- 2 tablespoons hemp seeds
- 4 walnuts
- 3 Brazil nuts
- 1 large banana
- 1 tablespoon extra-virgin coconut oil
- ½ cup unsweetened almond milk
- 1 cup water

Combine all of the ingredients in a blender. Blend on high speed until smooth, about 2 minutes. If the shake is too thick, add more water until you reach a thick but drinkable consistency. Serve chilled.

Nutritional analysis per serving (1 cup): calories 377, fat 17 g, saturated fat 3 g, cholesterol 0 mg, fiber 14 g, protein 12 g, carbohydrate 47 g, sodium 129 mg

BLUEBERRY MUFFINS

Serves: 6

Prep time: 10 minutes

Cook time: 30 minutes

Level: Easy

Budget: $

Yes, you can have muffins! Protein-rich almond meal is full of good mono-unsaturated and saturated fats; combined with eggs and berries, it provides a deprivation-free, protein-rich breakfast.

- 1 teaspoon extra-virgin olive oil
- 1 cup almond meal
- 2 teaspoons baking powder
- 2 teaspoons ground cinnamon
- ¼ teaspoon sea salt
- 4 large eggs
- 1 tablespoon unsweetened applesauce
- 1 tablespoon pure vanilla extract
- 1 cup frozen blueberries

1. Preheat the oven to 350°F. Line a 6-cup nonstick muffin pan with baking cups and lightly grease the cups with the oil.

2. Stir together the almond meal, baking powder, cinnamon, and salt in a large bowl.

3. In a separate small bowl, whisk together the eggs, applesauce, and vanilla extract.

4. Pour the wet ingredients into the dry ingredients and mix until there are no dry patches. Once the batter is smooth, fold in the blueberries.

5. Use a lightly greased 4-ounce ice cream scoop to divide the batter evenly among the 6 muffin cups. Give the pan a few gentle taps on the counter to remove any air bubbles that may be trapped in the batter.

6. Bake for 25–30 minutes. The muffins are cooked if a toothpick comes out clean when inserted into the center of a muffin. Let the muffins cool on a wire rack for 10 minutes before serving. Leftover muffins can be stored in the refrigerator for up to 2 days or in the freezer for up to 6 months.

Nutritional analysis per serving (1 muffin): calories 170, fat 12 g, saturated fat 2 g, cholesterol 109 mg, fiber 3 g, protein 8 g, carbohydrate 9 g, sodium 124 mg

BERRY BLAST CHIA PORRIDGE WITH HEMP MILK

This is a great example of a superfood! A no-grain porridge that will enlighten your palate and boost your metabolism. It's full of omega-3-rich anti-inflammatory compounds, hemp and chia seeds, magnesium, iron, and cinnamon, which help to balance blood sugar. It also tastes good, has great texture, and is full of protein and fiber. You can't go wrong!

- 1½ cups unsweetened almond milk
- 1 cup hemp seeds
- 1½ teaspoons ground cinnamon
- 1 teaspoon ground nutmeg
- 1½ teaspoons pure vanilla extract
- ½ cup extra-virgin olive oil
- 1 cup chia seeds
- 1 cup blueberries, for garnish
- 1 cup raspberries, for garnish
- 3 tablespoons cacao nibs, for garnish

Serves: 4

Prep time: 15 minutes

Level: Easy

Budget: $

1. Combine the almond milk, hemp seeds, cinnamon, nutmeg, vanilla, and olive oil in a blender. Blend on high speed until smooth, about 2 minutes.

2. Pour the blended hemp milk mixture into a large bowl and fold in the chia seeds. Garnish with fresh berries and cacao nibs. Leftover porridge can be stored in the refrigerator for up to 2 days but is best if served immediately.

Nutritional analysis per serving (½ cup): calories 327, fat 32 g, saturated fat 20 g, cholesterol 0 mg, fiber 7 g, protein 9 g, carbohydrate 11 g, sodium 14 mg

CHOCOLATE CHIA SEED PUDDING

Serves: 2

Prep time:
30 minutes

Level: Easy

Budget: $

Coconut, cacao, cayenne, and chia are all powerful superfoods that not only taste good but also reduce inflammation, help improve metabolism, and provide a rich source of omega-3 fats.

- ½ cup unsweetened coconut milk
- ¼ cup chia seeds
- 2 tablespoons extra-virgin coconut oil, melted
- 3 tablespoons unsweetened cacao powder
- 1 teaspoon pure vanilla extract
- ⅛ teaspoon cayenne pepper
- ⅛ teaspoon sea salt
- ¼ cup fresh blueberries, for garnish

1. Combine the coconut milk, chia seeds, and oil in a bowl and mix thoroughly. Let stand for 30 minutes on the counter.

2. Add the cacao, vanilla, cayenne pepper, and salt, and mix well. If the pudding is too thick, add a bit more coconut milk to thin it out. Garnish with the fresh berries. The pudding is best when served the same day.

Nutritional analysis per serving (½ cup): calories 226, fat 22 g, saturated fat 15 g, cholesterol 0 mg, fiber 8 g, protein 14 g, carbohydrate 11 g, sodium 88 mg

HEALTHIEST BREAKFAST IN THE WORLD

This is an easy breakfast containing seeds, nuts, spices, berries, antioxidants, and fiber. It tastes great and will keep you full. Green powders are typically freeze-dried superfoods such as wheat grass, spirulina, algae, broccoli or broccoli sprouts, spinach, and so on. They are added to smoothies and protein shakes to provide a nutrition boost. Hemp powder is the protein part of the plant extracted into a concentrated powder to provide a whole-foods, plant-based protein supplement often used in smoothies, shakes, and homemade snacks. Konjac powder is a natural source of soluble fiber from the konjac root plant found in China and Japan. The powder is used in smoothies and shakes to add bulk and lower the glycemic load of the meal. It slows absorption of fats and sugars into your bloodstream, reducing insulin and helping you lose weight and feel great.

Serves: 2

Prep time: 5 minutes

Level: Easy

Budget: $

- 2 tablespoons flaxseeds
- 1 tablespoon sesame seeds
- 2 teaspoons sunflower seeds
- 2 teaspoons pumpkin seeds
- 3 walnuts
- 5 almonds
- 1 tablespoon cacao powder
- 1 tablespoon green powder
- 2 tablespoons hemp protein powder
- 1 tablespoon konjac powder
- 1 teaspoon ground cinnamon
- ½ cup unsweetened coconut milk
- 1½ cups water, or as needed
- 8 strawberries, sliced
- ⅓ cup blueberries or sweet dark cherries

1. Place all of the seeds and nuts in a large spice grinder or coffee grinder. Grind for 1 minute until the mixture resembles coarse sand.
2. Transfer the ground seeds and nuts to a medium bowl. Add the cacao powder, green powder, hemp protein, konjac powder, cinnamon, and coconut milk and whisk until evenly mixed.

3. If it is too thick, mix in water as needed and stir until the mixture reaches a thick oatmeal consistency.

4. Fold in the strawberries and blueberries, reserving a few to scatter on top as a garnish. The mixture is best if eaten the same day.

Nutritional analysis per serving (½ cup): calories 276, fat 15 g, saturated fat 2 g, cholesterol 0 mg, fiber 13 g, protein 15 g, carbohydrate 25 g, sodium 17 mg

WEEKDAY VEGGIE SCRAMBLE

A simple veggie egg scramble is a great way to start the day. The eggs are a wonderful source of protein, and the extra omega-3 fats are anti-inflammatory and help reverse diabesity. Greens provide extra folate, magnesium, and B vitamins.

Serves: 2

Prep time: 5 minutes

Cook time: 10 minutes

Level: Easy

Budget: $

- 2 tablespoons extra virgin-olive oil
- ½ small red onion, finely chopped
- 2 garlic cloves, minced
- 1 large kale leaf, stemmed and roughly chopped
- ½ large red bell pepper, seeded and finely chopped
- 4 cremini mushrooms, thickly sliced
- sea salt and freshly ground black pepper
- 2 large eggs, beaten

1. Heat 1 tablespoon of the oil in a nonstick pan over medium-high heat. Once hot, add the onion and garlic. Cook for 1 minute while stirring constantly.

2. Toss in the kale and cook until it wilts and is bright green, about 3 minutes.

3. Add the bell pepper and mushrooms to the pan and season them to taste with salt and black pepper. Sauté the vegetables, stirring, until cooked through, 3–4 minutes. Transfer to a bowl and reserve.

4. Heat the remaining 1 tablespoon olive oil in the pan over low heat. Pour the eggs into the pan and stir constantly to scramble them. When the eggs look almost done—still the tiniest bit runny—fold the vegetables into the eggs, stirring, and cook for 1 more minute. Taste for seasoning, add more salt and black pepper if needed, and serve.

Nutritional analysis per serving (½ cup): calories 199, fat 18 g, saturated fat 3 g, cholesterol 164 mg, fiber 7 g, protein 14 g, carbohydrate 4 g, sodium 70 mg

GREEN EGG SKILLET BAKE

Serves: 4

Prep time: 10 minutes

Cook time: 20 minutes

Level: Easy

Budget: $

In this version of green eggs you won't even miss the ham. The flavorful olives stimulate your palate as the creamy tofu and coconut chili sauce nourish you. This is a fantastic breakfast—or enjoy it when you have "breakfast for dinner."

EGGS:

- 2 tablespoons extra-virgin olive oil
- 1 large Vidalia onion, thinly sliced
- sea salt and freshly ground black pepper
- 2 garlic cloves, minced
- ½ teaspoon ground turmeric
- 1 teaspoon ground cumin
- ½ teaspoon dried oregano
- ½ teaspoon red pepper flakes
- 1 small head collard greens, roughly chopped
- 4 cups baby spinach
- 8 cremini mushrooms, thickly sliced
- 4 large eggs

SAUCE:

- 2 tablespoons soft or silken tofu
- 1 tablespoon unsweetened coconut milk
- hot pepper sauce to taste
- ½ teaspoon red pepper flakes
- 1 garlic clove, minced
- sea salt and freshly ground black pepper

MAKE THE EGGS:

1. Preheat the oven to 400°F.

2. Heat 1 tablespoon of the olive oil in a large cast-iron pan over medium-high heat. Once hot, add the onion and season to taste with

salt and black pepper. Cook the onion until softened and golden, 5–6 minutes.

3. Add the garlic, turmeric, cumin, oregano, and red pepper flakes to the pan and cook with the onions for 2 minutes. Toss in the collard greens and cook, stirring constantly, until vibrant green, 3–4 minutes. Add the spinach and cook until wilted, about 2 minutes.

4. Turn off the heat and pour off any liquid that may have accumulated. Spread the vegetables into an even layer in the bottom of the pan. Scatter the sliced mushrooms over the vegetables.

5. Make four small wells in the vegetable mixture that are large enough to hold an egg comfortably. Crack an egg into each well, trying your best to not break the yolks. Season the tops of the eggs to taste with salt and black pepper and slide the pan into the oven.

6. Bake until the whites of the eggs are firm and the yolk is as cooked as you like, 7–10 minutes.

MAKE THE SAUCE:

While the eggs are baking, combine the tofu, coconut milk, hot pepper sauce, red pepper flakes, and garlic in a blender. Blend on high speed until smooth, and season the sauce to taste with salt and black pepper.

ASSEMBLE THE EGGS:

Pour a small amount of sauce over each egg. Drizzle the eggs with the remaining 1 tablespoon olive oil and serve family-style.

Nutritional analysis per serving (1 egg with veggies): calories 154, fat 9 g, saturated fat 1 g, cholesterol 53 mg, fiber 4 g, protein 6 g, carbohydrate 15 g, sodium 97 mg

VEGETABLE EGG SCRAMBLE

Serves: 1

Prep time:
10 minutes

Cook time:
5 minutes

Level: Easy

Budget: $

Omega-3-enriched eggs are a "functional food" readily available at your local supermarket. They come from chickens fed a diet rich in algae or flaxseeds, the original sources of these healthy fats.

- 2 large eggs
- 1 tablespoon water
- 1 teaspoon extra-virgin olive oil
- 1 cup assorted chopped raw vegetables (onions, red bell peppers, tomatoes, broccoli, zucchini, summer squash, asparagus, mushrooms, etc.)
- sea salt and freshly ground black pepper
- 2 tablespoons chunky tomato salsa

1. In a small bowl, whisk together the eggs and water until well mixed.
2. Heat the oil in a small cast-iron pan over medium heat. Add the vegetables and sauté until they are tender but still crisp, 2–3 minutes.
3. Pour the eggs over the vegetables and cook, stirring constantly, until the eggs scramble and set.
4. Season to taste with salt and black pepper, and top with the salsa.

Nutritional analysis per serving (2 cups): calories 202, fat 15 g, saturated fat 0 g, cholesterol 423 mg, fiber 1 g, protein 14 g, carbohydrate 4 g, sodium 144 mg

GARDEN OMELET

This superfood omelet contains many veggies that are detoxifying, anti-inflammatory, hormone-balancing, and nutrient-rich. Brussels sprouts and kale provide folate and glucosinolates, which help your body detoxify. Seaweeds are full of minerals and help bind heavy metals, avocados are loaded with healthy monounsaturated and saturated fats, and cilantro helps your body detoxify.

Serves: 4

Prep time: 10 minutes

Cook time: 20 minutes

Level: Easy

Budget: $

- sea salt
- 2 large kale leaves, stemmed and halved lengthwise
- 4 Brussels sprouts, trimmed and halved
- 3 large eggs
- 5 large egg whites
- freshly ground black pepper
- 2 tablespoons extra-virgin olive oil
- 6 cremini mushrooms, sliced
- ¼ cup chopped fresh cilantro
- ¼ cup chopped fresh dill
- 2 (½-ounce) packages roasted seaweed snacks (see note)
- 2 cups baby spinach
- 1 avocado, peeled, pitted, and sliced, for garnish
- 1 teaspoon white truffle oil (optional, for garnish)

1. Bring a large pot of water to a boil over high heat. When it boils, add a large pinch of salt. Drop in the kale leaves and Brussels sprouts and blanch just until they turn a brighter shade of green, 2–3 minutes. Drain well.

2. Crack the eggs into a medium mixing bowl, and add the other 5 egg whites. Beat the eggs and season to taste with salt and black pepper.

3. Heat the oil in a large nonstick pan over medium heat. Add the eggs and immediately turn the heat down to low. Stir to scramble the eggs, tilting the pan to distribute them in an even layer.

4. As soon as the eggs are no longer runny, arrange the Brussels sprouts on the left side of the omelet and scatter the mushrooms over them. Add a layer of kale and sprinkle the cilantro and dill on top. Cover the herbs with the seaweed and top with the spinach.

5. Cover the pan and cook over the lowest possible heat for 5 minutes.

6. Fold the omelet in half and then cut it into 4 sections. Garnish each portion with a few slices of avocado and drizzle on some truffle oil, if desired. The omelet should be eaten while hot.

Note: If you can't find roasted seaweed snacks, you can substitute 1 ounce plain nori. Before using, brush it with a tiny bit of oil and toast it in a lightly oiled skillet over medium heat for 10–15 seconds on each side. Cut into 3-inch squares before using in the omelet.

Nutritional analysis per serving (¼ omelet): calories 248, fat 18 g, saturated fat 3 g, cholesterol 123 mg, fiber 6 g, protein 14 g, carbohydrate 12 g, sodium 120 mg

ROASTED CHICKEN AND EGG WHITE CUP

This is like an egg muffin without the muffin! It's an unusual and delightful high-protein, vegetable-rich breakfast.

Serves: 12

Prep time: 15 minutes

Cook time: 30 minutes

Level: Easy

Budget: $

- 1 teaspoon extra-virgin olive oil
- 1 cup cooked chicken breast, roughly chopped
- 1 medium yellow bell pepper, seeded and finely chopped
- 2 cups baby spinach
- ½ bunch basil, finely chopped yielding about ½ ounce
- ½ large red onion, finely chopped
- 1 teaspoon red pepper flakes
- sea salt and freshly ground black pepper
- 12 large egg whites
- 2 tablespoons unsweetened soy milk
- 1 tablespoon Dijon mustard
- 2 garlic cloves, minced

1. Preheat the oven to 350°F. Lightly grease a 12-cup nonstick muffin pan with the oil and set aside.

2. In a large bowl stir together the chicken, bell pepper, spinach, basil, onion, ½ teaspoon of the red pepper flakes, and salt and black pepper to taste.

3. Combine the egg whites, soy milk, Dijon mustard, garlic, and ¼ teaspoon sea salt in a blender. Blend on medium speed for 2 minutes.

4. Fill each muffin cup with 3 tablespoons of the egg mixture and top with ¼ cup of the chicken and vegetable mixture. Season the top of each cup to taste with salt and the remaining ½ teaspoon red pepper flakes.

5. Put the pan in the oven on the middle rack and bake until the egg whites are puffed up and golden brown, 25–30 minutes.

6. Cool the pan on a wire rack for 5 minutes before serving. Any leftover cups can be stored in an airtight container and kept in the

refrigerator for up to 3 days. Reheat in a low oven or toaster oven before serving.

Nutritional analysis per serving (1 muffin cup): calories 57, fat 2 g, saturated fat 0 g, cholesterol 120 mg, fiber 1 g, protein 8 g, carbohydrate 2 g, sodium 120 mg

SOUPS

CURRIED CREAM OF CAULIFLOWER SOUP

Serves: 5

Prep time:
5 minutes

Cook time:
20 minutes

Level: Easy

Budget: $

This creamy, heartwarming soup contains curry powder (a powerful anti-inflammatory) and cauliflower (a powerful detoxifier), in a satisfying and delicious dairy-free blend.

- 3 cups low-sodium vegetable or chicken broth
- 1 cup unsweetened almond milk
- 1 large head cauliflower, cut into large florets
- 1 large carrot, peeled and chopped
- 1 tablespoon curry powder
- sea salt and freshly ground black pepper

1. Combine the broth, almond milk, vegetables, and curry powder in a medium pot and bring to a boil over high heat.

2. Once at a rolling boil, reduce the heat to low and cover the pot. Simmer until the cauliflower is tender but not mushy, about 15 minutes.

3. Take the pot off the heat and carefully transfer its contents to a blender. Blend on high until smooth and creamy. (Or use a handheld immersion blender to purée the soup right in the pot.) Taste for seasoning and adjust with salt and black pepper, if needed. Any leftover soup can be stored in the refrigerator for up to 4 days or in the freezer for up to 3 months.

Nutritional analysis per serving (1 cup): calories 50, fat 1 g, saturated fat 0 g, cholesterol 0 mg, fiber 3 g, protein 8 g, carbohydrate 438 g, sodium 543 mg

GREEN GODDESS BROCCOLI AND ARUGULA SOUP

Serves: 4

Prep time:
5 minutes

Cook time:
20 minutes

Level: Easy

Budget: $

Arugula and watercress are fabulous detoxifying foods full of vitamins and minerals. Combined with broccoli, these ingredients provide a healing, colorful, and vibrant soup. Lemon and arugula together create a peppery, tart, refreshing taste. Ghee is clarified butter used in South Asian cooking. Find it in Asian markets or natural foods stores.

- 1 teaspoon ghee
- ½ medium yellow onion, chopped
- 2 garlic cloves, finely chopped
- 1 large head broccoli, cut into medium florets
- 1 cup arugula
- 2½ cups low-sodium vegetable broth
- ½ cup unsweetened coconut milk
- juice of ½ lemon, or more if needed
- sea salt and freshly ground black pepper

1. Heat the ghee in a medium pot over medium-high heat. Once melted, add the onion and garlic and cook until aromatic and soft, about 3 minutes.

2. Add the broccoli and arugula to the pan and stir frequently until the broccoli is bright green and the arugula has wilted, 4–5 minutes.

3. Pour in the broth and bring the soup to a boil.

4. Once boiling, reduce the heat to low and simmer until the broccoli is fully cooked, 5–8 minutes.

5. Carefully transfer the soup to a blender and blend on high speed for 1½ minutes. Pour in the coconut milk and lemon juice and blend for another 30 seconds. (Or use a handheld immersion blender to purée the soup right in the pot.) Taste for seasoning and adjust with salt, black pepper, and lemon juice if needed. The soup should be thick but still light. If it is too thick, thin it with a little more coconut milk

or water. Any leftover soup can be stored in the refrigerator for up to 5 days or in the freezer for up to 6 months.

Nutritional analysis per serving (1¼ cups): calories 104, fat 4 g, saturated fat 1 g, cholesterol 0 mg, fiber 5 g, protein 5 g, carbohydrate 13 g, sodium 289 mg

CREAMY ASPARAGUS SOUP

Serves: 6

Prep time: 10 minutes

Cook time: 25 minutes

Level: Easy

Budget: $

Asparagus, one of my favorite foods, can be eaten in unlimited quantities. This creamy soup is full of folate and antioxidants.

- 1 tablespoon extra-virgin olive oil
- 3 garlic cloves, minced
- 1 head cauliflower, cut into small florets
- 2½ pounds asparagus, trimmed
- ¼ teaspoon cayenne pepper
- sea salt and freshly ground black pepper
- 6 cups low-sodium vegetable or chicken broth, or water

1. Heat the oil in a medium pot over medium-high heat. After a minute, add the garlic and cook for 1 minute.

2. Put the cauliflower and asparagus in the pot, add the cayenne pepper, and season to taste with salt and black pepper. Cook for 4–5 minutes, stirring frequently.

3. Pour in the broth and bring the soup to a boil, then reduce the heat to low and simmer until the cauliflower is fully cooked, 5–8 minutes.

4. Carefully transfer the soup to a blender and blend on high speed until smooth, about 2 minutes. (Or use a handheld immersion blender to purée the soup directly in the pot.) Taste for seasoning and adjust with salt and black pepper if needed. The soup should be thick but still light. If it is too thick, thin it with a little more broth or water. Any leftover soup can be stored in the refrigerator for up to 5 days or in the freezer for up to 6 months.

Nutritional analysis per serving (1 cup): calories 99, fat 4 g, saturated fat 0 g, cholesterol 0 mg, fiber 7 g, protein 6 g, carbohydrate 14 g, sodium 224 mg

Brazilian Black Bean Soup

The smokiness from the cumin gives this black bean soup a unique flavor. If you like it hot, you can add extra red pepper flakes. Enjoy this soup all week long and enjoy excellent digestion.

Serves: 4

Prep time: 10 minutes

Cook time: 35 minutes

Level: Easy

Budget: $

- 1 tablespoon extra-virgin olive oil
- 2 celery ribs, finely chopped
- 1 small yellow onion, finely chopped
- 1 garlic clove, minced
- ½ small poblano pepper, seeded and finely chopped
- 2 cups low-sodium vegetable broth
- 2 cups cooked black beans or 1 (15-ounce) can black beans, rinsed and drained
- 2 teaspoons chili powder
- ⅛ teaspoon ground cloves
- 1 teaspoon ground cumin
- ¼ teaspoon paprika
- ⅛ teaspoon red pepper flakes
- sea salt to taste
- 3 tablespoons chopped fresh cilantro, for garnish

1. Heat the oil in a medium pot over medium heat. Sauté the celery, onion, garlic, and pepper until the vegetables start to soften, 4–5 minutes.

2. Add the broth, beans, and all of the spices to the pot and stir until well mixed. Bring to a boil, then simmer for 10 minutes, stirring occasionally, until the flavors come together.

3. Add the cilantro and simmer for an additional minute. Serve immediately. Any leftover black bean soup can be refrigerated for up to 5 days or frozen for up to 4 months.

Nutritional analysis per serving (1 cup): calories 171, fat 22 g, saturated fat 0 g, cholesterol 0 mg, fiber 9 g, protein 10 g, carbohydrate 29 g, sodium 771 mg

CURRIED GREAT NORTHERN BEAN AND CARROT SOUP

Serves: 4

Prep time:
10 minutes

Cook time:
30 minutes

Level: Easy

Budget: $

Curry is one of the most prized spice mixes in the world because of its beautiful color and unique aroma. It is just as healthy as it is beautiful—the turmeric in curry is a potent anti-inflammatory phytonutrient.

- 1 tablespoon extra-virgin olive oil
- 3 medium carrots, peeled and thinly sliced
- 1 small yellow onion, chopped
- 1 garlic clove, minced
- 1 medium shallot, minced
- 1-inch piece fresh ginger, peeled and minced
- 2 cups low-sodium vegetable broth
- 2 cups cooked Great Northern beans or 1 (15-ounce) can Great Northern beans, rinsed and drained
- ⅛ teaspoon curry powder
- ⅛ teaspoon cayenne pepper
- sea salt and freshly ground black pepper
- juice of ½ lemon

1. Heat the oil in a medium pot over medium heat. Sauté the carrots, onion, garlic, shallot, and ginger until the vegetables start to soften, 4–6 minutes.
2. Add the broth, beans, curry powder, and cayenne pepper. Turn the heat to high and bring the soup to a boil.
3. When it boils, cover the pot and reduce the heat to low. Simmer the soup until the carrots are very tender, 15–20 minutes. Remove the pot from the heat and season to taste with salt and black pepper.
4. Transfer the soup to a blender, add the lemon juice, and blend on high speed until smooth, about 2 minutes. (Or use a handheld immersion blender to purée the soup directly in the pot.) Serve immediately.

Any leftover soup can be refrigerated for up to 5 days or frozen for up to 4 months.

Nutritional analysis per serving (1 cup): calories 116, fat 41 g, saturated fat 1 g, cholesterol 0 mg, fiber 3 g, protein 4 g, carbohydrate 16 g, sodium 301 mg

TUSCAN ZUCCHINI SOUP

Serves: 4

Prep time:
10 minutes

Cook time:
10 minutes

Level: Easy

Budget: $

For a nourishing, low-glycemic soup, try this wonderful Tuscan recipe. It's inexpensive—and a great way to use up zucchini from the garden.

- 4 large zucchini, quartered
- ½ cup extra-virgin olive oil
- juice of ½ small lemon, or more if needed
- 1 garlic clove, minced
- ½ bunch fresh basil (about ½ ounce)
- sea salt and freshly ground black pepper
- 1 tomato, finely chopped

1. Put the zucchini in a large pot and add water to cover. Bring to a boil over high heat. Reduce the heat to medium-low and cook at a brisk simmer until tender, 8–10 minutes.

2. Drain the zucchini and reserve ½ cup of the cooking liquid. Transfer the zucchini to a blender and blend on high speed until smooth, about 1 minute. While the blender is running, add the olive oil, reserved cooking liquid, lemon juice, garlic, half of the basil, and salt and black pepper to taste. Blend for another minute until well mixed and check for seasoning; adjust with lemon juice, salt, and black pepper if needed.

3. Garnish each serving with some chopped tomato and a few basil leaves. The soup is best served hot or at room temperature. Leftover zucchini soup can be refrigerated for up to 5 days; reblend and reheat the soup before serving.

Nutritional analysis per serving (1 cup): calories 253, fat 27 g, saturated fat 0 g, cholesterol 0 mg, fiber 1 g, protein 1 g, carbohydrate 3 g, sodium 243 mg

Tuscan White Bean Stew

Mirepoix is an aromatic flavor foundation for soups, broths, and sauces. It comes from the French culinary tradition and is usually made from carrots, onions, and celery. Enjoy the taste of these delicious vegetables in this stew.

- 1 tablespoon extra-virgin olive oil
- 1 small yellow onion, finely chopped
- 2 medium carrots, peeled and finely chopped
- 1 garlic clove, minced
- 2 celery ribs, finely chopped
- sea salt and freshly ground black pepper
- 2 cups low-sodium vegetable broth
- 2 cup cooked Great Northern beans or 1 (15-ounce) can Great Northern beans, rinsed and drained
- 1 teaspoon chopped fresh parsley
- ½ teaspoon chopped fresh rosemary
- ½ teaspoon chopped fresh thyme

Serves: 4
Prep time: 10 minutes
Cook time: 35 minutes
Level: Easy
Budget: $

1. Heat the oil in a medium pot over medium heat and sauté the onions until fragrant, 2–3 minutes.

2. Add the carrots, garlic, and celery, season the vegetables to taste with salt and black pepper, and cook until soft, 4–5 minutes.

3. Add the vegetable broth, beans, and fresh herbs. Bring the soup to a boil, reduce the heat to low, and cover the pot. Simmer for 20–30 minutes, stirring the soup occasionally.

4. Remove the pot from the heat and serve. Any leftover soup can be stored in the refrigerator for up to 5 days or in the freezer for up to 4 months.

Nutritional analysis per serving (1 cup): calories 106, fat 16 g, saturated fat 0 g, cholesterol 0 mg, fiber 4 g, protein 5 g, carbohydrate 18 g, sodium 874 mg

Serves: 6

Prep time:
15 minutes

Cook time:
10 minutes

Level: Easy

Budget: $

SALADS

SPICED TURKEY SALAD

Spices are a wonderful way to enhance both the flavor and the medicinal power of your meal. Paprika, cumin, black pepper, garlic, and cilantro all have unique chemical healing ingredients designed to boost your metabolism—and delight your palate.

- 1 pound lean ground turkey
- 1 teaspoon smoked paprika
- ½ teaspoon ground cumin
- 1 teaspoon garlic powder
- ¼ teaspoon freshly ground black pepper
- ½ teaspoon sea salt
- 2 tablespoons extra-virgin olive oil
- 5 ounces spring salad mix
- 2 cups cooked black beans or 1 (15-ounce) can black beans, rinsed and drained
- 4 medium tomatoes, roughly chopped
- ¼ cup chopped fresh cilantro

1. Combine the turkey and all of the seasonings in a medium bowl and mix well. Let the turkey mixture sit for 10–15 minutes.
2. Heat the oil in a medium cast iron-pan over medium–high heat. Once hot, add the turkey. Cook, breaking up the meat with a fork, until it is browned and crumbly, about 8 minutes. Remove the turkey from the pan and let it cool fully.
3. In a large bowl, mix the greens, beans, and tomatoes. Scatter the turkey across the top of the salad and sprinkle on the cilantro. This salad is best if eaten the same day. If there are any leftovers, store the

turkey separately from the greens and combine before serving. The cooked turkey can be refrigerated for up to 3 days.

Nutritional analysis per serving (1 cup): calories 235, fat 11 g, saturated fat 2 g, cholesterol 54 mg, fiber 5 g, protein 20 g, carbohydrate 14 g, sodium 106 mg

BLACK BEAN SALAD

Serves: 4

Prep time:
10 minutes

Cook time:
30 minutes

Level: Easy

Budget: $

Caramelizing the onions is the secret to this dish. Let the onions cook down to deepen the flavor of this pungent and tasty salad.

DRESSING:

- juice of 2 small lemons
- ½ teaspoon chopped fresh oregano
- ¼ teaspoon ground cumin
- ¼ teaspoon cayenne pepper
- 3 tablespoons extra-virgin olive oil
- sea salt and freshly ground black pepper

SALAD:

- 1 tablespoon extra-virgin olive oil
- 2 large red onions, finely chopped
- 2 large yellow onions, finely chopped
- 1 small jalapeño pepper, seeded and minced
- 5 garlic cloves, minced
- 2 cups cooked black beans or 1 (15-ounce) can black beans, rinsed and drained
- 2 scallions (white parts only), thinly sliced
- 1 large carrot, peeled and finely chopped
- 2 celery ribs, diced

MAKE THE DRESSING:

In a small bowl whisk together the lemon juice, oregano, and spices until evenly mixed. Slowly pour in the oil while whisking until the dressing has thickened and emulsified. Check the dressing for seasoning and add salt and black pepper to taste.

MAKE THE SALAD:

1. Heat the oil in a large sauté pan over medium heat. After a minute add the onions and sauté until they release all their moisture, 5–6

minutes. Turn the heat to low and continue to cook the onions until they are brown and caramelized, 15–20 minutes. Stir frequently so that the onions cook evenly and don't burn.

2. Add the jalapeño and garlic and cook until the garlic browns slightly, about 5 minutes. Transfer the vegetable mixture to a large bowl and set aside to cool.

3. When cool, add the beans, scallions, carrot, and celery to the caramelized onion mixture and mix well.

ASSEMBLE THE SALAD:

Pour the dressing over the black bean mixture and gently mix until the dressing thoroughly covers the beans. Serve. Store in a glass container in the refrigerator for up to 3 days.

Nutritional analysis per serving (1 cup): calories 272, fat 91, saturated fat 1 g, cholesterol 0 mg, fiber 12 g, protein 12 g, carbohydrate 36 g, sodium 20 mg

GRAPEFRUIT AND AVOCADO SALAD WITH DIJON LIME VINAIGRETTE

Serves: 4

Prep time: 15 minutes

Level: Easy

Budget: $

The lime, cilantro, and mustard spice up the lettuce and avocado, making this a light, cleansing, detoxifying, and alkalinizing salad.

DIJON LIME VINAIGRETTE:

- 1 tablespoon apple cider vinegar
- ½ teaspoon Dijon mustard
- juice of 1 lime
- ¼ cup extra-virgin olive oil
- sea salt and freshly ground black pepper to taste

SALAD:

- 2 heads butter lettuce, leaves separated
- ½ cup chopped fresh cilantro
- 1 large grapefruit, peeled and segmented
- 1 avocado, peeled, pitted, and sliced
- ½ small red onion, finely sliced

MAKE THE VINAIGRETTE:

Combine all of the vinaigrette ingredients in a blender and blend on high for 30 seconds.

ASSEMBLE THE SALAD:

Spoon a few tablespoons of vinaigrette around the sides of a large salad bowl. Add the lettuce and cilantro and toss to coat them lightly and evenly with vinaigrette. Arrange the lettuce and cilantro on a platter forming a bed. Scatter the grapefruit, avocado, and onion over the lettuce and drizzle on as much vinaigrette as you like. Leftover vinaigrette can be stored in the refrigerator for up to 5 days.

Nutritional analysis per serving (1 cup): calories 197, fat 18 g, saturated fat 3 g, cholesterol 0 mg, fiber 5 g, protein 2 g, carbohydrate 10 g, sodium 78 mg

STRAWBERRY SPINACH SALAD

Macadamia nuts and strawberries are a wonderful combination. This salad is cool and refreshing, great for a summer party.

VINAIGRETTE:

- 10 fresh strawberries, hulled
- 2 tablespoons balsamic vinegar
- 2 tablespoons sesame seeds
- ½ cup extra-virgin olive oil
- ¼ teaspoon sea salt
- ¼ teaspoon freshly ground black pepper

SALAD:

- 5 ounces baby spinach
- ¼ small red onion, thinly sliced
- ¼ cup chopped toasted macadamia nuts
- 14 fresh strawberries, hulled and thinly sliced

MAKE THE VINAIGRETTE:

Combine all of the vinaigrette ingredients in a blender and blend on high speed for 30 seconds. Check for seasoning and add more salt and black pepper if needed.

ASSEMBLE THE SALAD:

In a large bowl combine the spinach, onion, macadamia nuts, and strawberries and toss gently. Serve the vinaigrette on the side. Leftover vinaigrette can be stored in the refrigerator for up to 5 days.

Nutritional analysis per serving (½ cup): calories 235, fat 24 g, saturated fat 3 g, cholesterol 0 mg, fiber 2 g, protein 2 g, carbohydrate 6 g, sodium 123 mg

Serves: 6
Prep time: 10 minutes
Level: Easy
Budget: $$

DR. HYMAN'S RAW KALE SALAD

Serves: 4

Prep time:
10 minutes

Level: Easy

Budget: $

Massaging finely chopped kale with lemon and olive oil breaks down the kale's stiffness and bitterness, leaving you with tender greens bursting with flavor. Don't skimp on the chopping! Not having to chew through large pieces of raw kale increases your eating pleasure.

- 1 large bunch kale, stemmed and finely chopped
- zest and juice of 1 large lemon
- ¼ cup extra-virgin olive oil
- 1 garlic clove, minced
- ⅛ teaspoon sea salt
- ¼ cup toasted pine nuts
- ¼ cup currants
- ½ cup chopped pitted kalamata olives

1. Place the kale in a large salad bowl and add the lemon zest and juice, olive oil, garlic, and salt. Massage the mixture with your hands for 1–2 minutes to soften the kale.

2. Add the remaining ingredients and toss to combine.

3. Allow the salad to rest and soften for about 15 minutes before serving. Kale salad is best if eaten the same day but can be stored overnight in the refrigerator.

Nutritional analysis per serving (1 cup): calories 227, fat 21 g, saturated fat 3 g, cholesterol 0 mg, fiber 3 g, protein 4 g, carbohydrate 11 g, sodium 234 mg

CILANTRO, EDAMAME, AND PINE NUT SALAD

Plant proteins are important in reversing diabesity. The creamy cilantro dressing is a luxurious finish to this soybean salad.

Serves: 4

Prep time: 20 minutes

Cook time: 5 minutes

Level: Easy

Budget: $

DRESSING:

- ⅓ cup Vegenaise or mayonnaise
- ⅓ cup chopped fresh cilantro
- juice of 1 lime, or more if needed
- ¼ teaspoon sea salt
- freshly ground black pepper to taste

SALAD:

- 1 (10-ounce) bag frozen soybeans, thawed
- 2 small carrots, peeled and grated
- ½ small red onion, finely chopped
- ½ large red bell pepper, seeded and finely chopped
- 1 celery rib, finely chopped
- ¼ cup sunflower seeds
- 5 ounces mixed salad greens
- ¼ cup pine nuts, for garnish

MAKE THE DRESSING:

In a small bowl, whisk together all of the dressing ingredients until smooth. Check for seasoning and adjust if needed with additional lime juice, salt, and black pepper.

ASSEMBLE THE SALAD:

1. In a medium bowl, combine the soybeans, carrots, red onion, bell pepper, celery, and sunflower seeds.
2. Spoon some dressing onto the salad and toss gently to coat. Add as much dressing as you like.

197

3. Lay the greens on a platter and pour the soybean mixture over them. Garnish with the pine nuts. Any leftover soybean mixture or dressing can be stored in the refrigerator for up to 4 days.

Nutritional analysis per serving (1 cup): calories 189, fat 14 g, saturated fat 1 g, cholesterol 0 mg, fiber 4 g, protein 6 g, carbohydrate 12 g, sodium 187 mg

ENTRÉES

PAM'S DELICIOUS AND HEALTHY VEGETABLE STIR-FRY

Serves: 2

Prep time: 5 minutes

Cook time: 20 minutes

Level: Easy

Budget: $

Stir-fries are a fun, easy way to take leftovers from the refrigerator and make a wonderful dish. You can combine many different ingredients, including tofu and seasonal vegetables, in a simple sauté to help you fill up and feel good.

- 1 tablespoon extra-virgin coconut oil
- 4 ounces firm tofu, drained, pressed, and cut into 1-inch cubes
- ½ teaspoon sea salt
- 2 garlic cloves, minced
- ½ teaspoon red pepper flakes
- ½ medium red onion, finely chopped
- 8 shiitake mushrooms, stemmed and thickly sliced
- ¼ head cauliflower, cut into small florets
- 3 asparagus spears, trimmed and thinly sliced
- ¼ cup chopped fresh basil
- 1 teaspoon liquid amino acids, such as Bragg's (optional)

1. Heat 1 teaspoon of the oil in a wok or large cast-iron pan over medium-high heat. When hot, add the tofu and ¼ teaspoon of the salt and stir-fry until evenly brown, 3–4 minutes. Add the garlic and red pepper flakes and cook with the tofu for 2 minutes, stirring constantly so that the garlic doesn't burn. Transfer the tofu and garlic to a plate and set aside.

2. Put the pan back over medium-high heat and add the remaining 2 teaspoons oil. Add the onion to the pan and stir-fry until soft, 2–3 minutes. Add the mushrooms, cauliflower, and asparagus and season the vegetables with the remaining ¼ teaspoon salt. Cook, stirring frequently, until the cauliflower is just cooked through, 6–8 minutes.

3. Turn off the heat and sprinkle in the basil and amino acids, if desired. Add the reserved tofu and garlic back to the pan and toss everything together.

4. Pour the stir-fry out onto a platter and serve while hot. Any leftover stir-fry can be refrigerated for up to 4 days.

Nutritional analysis per serving (1 cup): calories 182, fat 10 g, saturated fat 2 g, cholesterol 0 mg, fiber 8 g, protein 8 g, carbohydrate 17 g, sodium 438 mg

SPICY TRIPLE GREEN SAUTÉ

Serves: 3

Prep time: 10 minutes

Cook time: 30 minutes

Level: Easy

Budget: $

Greens, mushrooms, and a spicy tomato sauce make a great stir-fry. This dish is delicious and has powerful healing properties. Enjoy.

SPICY SAUCE:

- 1 tablespoon extra-virgin olive oil
- 1 tablespoon red pepper flakes
- 2 garlic cloves, minced
- 1 (16-ounce can) diced tomatoes, drained
- sea salt and freshly ground black pepper

GREENS:

- 2 tablespoons grapeseed oil
- ½ large red onion, thinly sliced
- 4 garlic cloves, minced
- 4 ounces shiitake mushrooms, stemmed and sliced
- 1 large bunch Swiss chard, stemmed and chopped
- 1 large bunch mustard greens, stemmed and chopped
- 1 large bunch beet greens, stemmed and chopped
- sea salt and freshly ground black pepper

MAKE THE SPICY SAUCE:

1. Heat the olive oil in a medium saucepan over medium heat. Add the red pepper flakes and garlic to the hot oil and stir frequently for 30 seconds. Pour in the tomatoes and season the mixture to taste with salt and black pepper.

2. Reduce the heat to low, cover the pan, and simmer the sauce for 15–20 minutes. Remove from the heat and set aside.

MAKE THE GREENS:

1. Heat the grapeseed oil in a wok or large cast-iron pan. When hot, add the onion and garlic and stir-fry for 1–2 minutes. Add the mushrooms

to the pan and cook them for a few minutes, just until they've begun to soften and give off their liquid.

2. Toss in the greens and cook until bright green, 6–8 minutes.

3. Pour in the spicy sauce and cook until the sauce has thickened slightly, 6-8 minutes. Season to taste with salt and black pepper, pour the greens out onto a platter, and serve hot. Leftover greens can be refrigerated for up to 5 days.

Nutritional analysis per serving (1⅓ cups): calories 177, fat 9 g, saturated fat 1 g, cholesterol 0 mg, fiber 7 g, protein 4 g, carbohydrate 21 g, sodium 229 mg

MIGHTY "MEATY" MEATLESS STEW

You won't believe how the combination of eggplant and mushrooms can create a meaty mouthful! This stew is real comfort food—hearty and full of a variety of herbs and one secret ingredient (anchovies!), which lends smokiness and a touch of salty-savory to the overall dish. Be sure to finish it off with a fresh herb such as parsley, to add a hint of freshness to this filling meal.

Serves: 10

Prep time: 15 minutes

Cook time: 30 minutes

Level: Easy

Budget: $

- 2 tablespoons extra-virgin olive oil
- 1 (2-ounce) can olive oil–packed anchovies, drained
- 1 large Vidalia onion, chopped
- 5 garlic cloves, minced
- 4 celery ribs, sliced ½-inch thick
- 2 large carrots, peeled and sliced ½-inch thick
- 2 tablespoons dried parsley
- 1 tablespoon dried marjoram
- 1 tablespoon dried basil
- 1 tablespoon fennel seed
- 1 tablespoon red pepper flakes
- sea salt and freshly ground black pepper to taste
- 1 large eggplant, peeled and finely chopped
- 5 cups mushrooms (about 1 pound), thickly sliced
- 2 medium zucchini, halved lengthwise and thickly sliced crosswise
- 2 (12-ounce) jars hot or sweet cherry or banana peppers, drained and sliced
- 2 (28-ounce) cans crushed tomatoes
- 1 cup low-sodium chicken broth
- ¼ cup dry red wine
- 1 large bunch kale, stemmed and roughly chopped
- 1 cup water
- 4 cups cooked red kidney beans or 2 (15-ounce) cans kidney beans, rinsed and drained
- ¼ large head cauliflower, cut into medium florets
- 1 cup pitted and halved small black olives
- ½ cup chopped fresh parsley, for garnish

1. Heat the oil in a large pot over medium heat. When hot, add the anchovies, onion, garlic, celery, carrots, dried parsley, marjoram, basil, and fennel seed. Stir well and cook until the onions are soft, 5–6 minutes. Season with the red pepper flakes and salt and black pepper to taste, and mix until the anchovies melt into the vegetables and disappear.

2. Add the eggplant, mushrooms, and zucchini and cook until they're tender but still firm, about 5 minutes.

3. Toss in the hot or sweet peppers and pour in the tomatoes, broth, and wine. Raise the heat to high and bring to a boil.

4. Reduce the heat to medium-low and add the kale and the water. Let the kale simmer until it wilts, 2–3 minutes. Add the beans, cauliflower, and olives and continue to simmer, 5–7 minutes. If the stew is very thick, loosen it up with a little more broth or water.

5. Check the stew for seasoning and add additional salt and black pepper if desired. Garnish the stew with the parsley and serve. Any leftovers can be stored in the refrigerator for up to 5 days or in the freezer for up to 6 months.

Nutritional analysis per serving (2 cups): calories 321, fat 7 g, saturated fat 1 g, cholesterol 147 mg, fiber 12 g, protein 27 g, carbohydrate 38 g, sodium 328 mg

Vegan Lasagna

Eating healthy foods does not have to be about deprivation. This fabulous vegan lasagna proves that it can be good *and* good for you. The combination of wonderful vegetables and protein is both healthful and satisfying.

MACADAMIA "MOZZARELLA CHEESE":

- 1 cup raw macadamia nuts
- 2 teaspoons white miso
- ½ teaspoon garlic powder
- ½ teaspoon sea salt
- ¾ cup water

CASHEW "PARMESAN CHEESE":

- ½ cup raw cashews
- 2 garlic cloves, finely chopped
- 1 teaspoon sea salt

TOMATO SAUCE:

- 1 tablespoon extra-virgin olive oil
- 4 garlic cloves, finely chopped
- 1 small red onion, finely chopped
- 1 bay leaf
- 1 teaspoon dried oregano
- 1 tablespoon balsamic vinegar
- 6 plum tomatoes, roughly chopped
- sea salt and freshly ground black pepper

SPINACH VERDE SAUCE:

- 3 cups baby spinach
- ½ red bell pepper, seeded and chopped
- ½ cup water
- sea salt and freshly ground black pepper to taste

Serves: 8
Prep time: 1 hour
Cook time: 2 hours
Level: Difficult
Budget: $$

VEGETABLES:

- 3 tablespoons extra-virgin olive oil
- 1 large eggplant, thinly sliced
- 2 large zucchini, thinly sliced

MAKE THE "CHEESES":

1. Place all of the macadamia "mozzarella" ingredients in a blender. Blend on high speed until creamy and smooth, 2–3 minutes. Transfer to a bowl and set aside.

2. Place all of the cashew "Parmesan" ingredients in a food processor. Pulse until close to the consistency of grated Parmesan cheese. Transfer to a bowl and set aside.

MAKE THE TOMATO SAUCE:

Heat the oil in a medium pot over medium-high heat. Add the garlic and the onion and sauté until aromatic, 3–4 minutes. Stir in the bay leaf, oregano, balsamic vinegar, and tomatoes and season to taste with salt and black pepper. Cover the pan and simmer the sauce over low heat for 30 minutes. Remove the bay leaf once done.

MAKE THE SPINACH VERDE SAUCE:

Combine all of the spinach verde sauce ingredients in a blender and blend on high speed until smooth, about 2 minutes. Transfer to a bowl and set aside.

ASSEMBLE THE LASAGNA:

1. Preheat the oven to 375°F. Grease a 9 x 13-inch baking dish with 1 tablespoon of the oil and begin layering the components. Start with a layer of one-fourth of the eggplant and zucchini slices at the bottom, and then spread all of the spinach verde sauce on top in an even layer. Add another layer of eggplant and zucchini and spoon on half of the tomato sauce. Then add another layer of eggplant and zucchini and sprinkle with the macadamia "mozzarella." Add the last layer of egg-

plant and zucchini and top with the remaining half of the tomato sauce.

2. Sprinkle the cashew "Parmesan" over the top and lightly drizzle the lasagna with the remaining 2 tablespoons olive oil. Cover with foil and bake for 45 minutes.

3. Remove the foil and bake, uncovered, until the top of the lasagna is golden brown, about 45 minutes more.

4. Let cool for 10 minutes and then serve. Any leftover lasagna can be stored in the refrigerator for up to 4 days or in the freezer for up to 4 months.

Nutritional analysis per serving (1 cup): calories 249, fat 21 g, saturated fat 3 g, cholesterol 0 mg, fiber 6 g, protein 5 g, carbohydrate 16 g, sodium 242 mg

MOM'S POACHED FISH IN VELVETY TOMATO SAUCE

Serves 4

Prep time:
10 minutes

Cook time:
30 minutes

Level: Easy

Budget: $

The spices in this dish lend dimension to the tangy tomatoes and create a warming and luscious broth to accompany the fish. You can use halibut or any firm white fish if you can't find cod. This is particularly tasty served over steamed or lightly sautéed kale or Swiss chard.

- 2 tablespoons extra-virgin olive oil
- 1 medium yellow onion, finely chopped
- 1 garlic clove, minced
- ½-inch piece fresh ginger, peeled and grated
- 1 (15 ounce) can fire-roasted chopped tomatoes
- sea salt and freshly ground black pepper to taste
- ½ teaspoon curry powder (optional)
- 1½ pounds fresh firm, white fish (cod, halibut, haddock), cut into 3-inch pieces
- ½ cup chopped fresh parsley, for garnish
- 2 bunches kale, rinsed and chopped

1. Heat the olive oil in a large saucepan over medium-low heat. Sauté the onion until translucent, 5–7 minutes, then add the garlic, ginger, tomatoes, salt, black pepper, and curry powder, if desired. Cook for 20 minutes, stirring occasionally.

2. Add the fish, cover, and cook until opaque, 8–10 minutes. Be careful not to overcook. The fish will add its own liquid to the dish. Sprinkle with fresh parsley and serve. Leftover fish in tomato sauce can be refrigerated for up to 2 days.

Nutritional analysis per serving (4 ounces fish, 1 cup kale): calories 258, fat 9 g, saturated fat 1 g, cholesterol 62 mg, fiber 3 g, protein 30 g, carbohydrate 16 g, sodium 310 mg

Pesce al Cartoccio (Fish Baked in Parchment Paper)

This is a delightful way to steam light fish, leaving it soft, tender, flaky, and flavorful.

Serves: 8

Prep time: 5 minutes

Cook time: 25 minutes

Level: Easy

Budget: $$

- 4 (8-ounce) salmon or halibut fillets
- 3 tablespoons extra-virgin olive oil
- juice and zest of 1 lemon
- sea salt and freshly ground pepper
- 4 medium tomatoes, thinly sliced
- 1 large orange, thinly sliced
- 3 scallions (white parts only), finely chopped
- 8 fresh basil leaves, finely sliced
- 8 fresh thyme sprigs
- 1 tablespoon capers, rinsed and drained
- 1 cup dry white wine, such as Chardonnay

1. Preheat the oven to 400°F.
2. Place four 18-inch circles of parchment paper on a work surface and brush them lightly with ½ tablespoon of the oil. Fold each circle in half and then unfold it. Lay the fish, skin-side down, next to the crease.
3. Brush each fillet with ½ tablespoon olive oil, sprinkle with the lemon zest, and season to taste with salt and black pepper.
4. Lay two slices of tomato and two slices of orange on each piece of fish and brush the lemon juice over the fillets. Top with the scallions, herbs, and capers.
5. Start to fold the parchment. Your goal is to make a tightly sealed pouch for the fish to steam in. Start by folding the parchment at the line you created earlier so that the two sides of paper meet to form a half circle. Then, starting at the rounded bottom of the half circle, begin to make ½-inch folds, sealing each fold as tightly as possible. You should eventually have a half-moon shape with small pleats all

around the edge and a little air pocket where the fish is. Before you make the last fold to seal the end of the packet, pour ¼ cup of wine into the unsealed part of each packet. Make the last folds to seal the fish in, being careful not to spill the wine while doing so.

6. Brush the top of the parchment lightly with the remaining ½ tablespoon oil. This will prevent the paper from completely charring during the cooking. Place the parchment pockets on a baking sheet and slide them into the oven on the top rack. Bake for 10 minutes per inch of thickness of fish.

7. When done, carefully unwrap or cut the parchment with a knife or scissors. Open carefully, as the escaping steam will be very hot. Serve the fish in its own wrapping or remove and plate each portion.

Nutritional analysis per serving (½ fillet): calories 286, fat 18 g, saturated fat 3 g, cholesterol 71 mg, fiber 1 g, protein 26 g, carbohydrate 3 g, sodium 253 mg

BAKED COD WITH THYME

Using herbs to crust your fish is a flavorful and healthy way to add a hint of elegance to your weeknight meal. Complete this dish with a squeeze of fresh lemon.

- 1 tablespoon plus 1 teaspoon extra-virgin olive oil
- 1 teaspoon fresh thyme, minced
- ½ teaspoon sea salt
- ¼ teaspoon onion powder
- 4 (6-ounce) skinless cod fillets

Serves: 4

Prep time: 5 minutes

Cook time: 15 minutes

Level: Easy

Budget: $$

1. Preheat the oven to 375°F. Grease a baking sheet with 1 teaspoon of the oil and set aside.

2. Combine the remaining 1 tablespoon oil, thyme, salt, and onion powder in a bowl and stir until mixed well.

3. Season the cod fillets evenly with the spice mixture and place them on the baking sheet.

4. Put the pan in the oven on the top rack and bake until the fish flakes easily with a fork, 12–15 minutes.

5. Transfer to a platter and serve. Leftover fish can be refrigerated for up to 2 days.

Nutritional analysis per serving (1 fillet): calories 232, fat 7 g, saturated fat 1 g, cholesterol 98 mg, fiber 0 g, protein 40 g, carbohydrate 0 g, sodium 250 mg

COD WITH ROASTED CHILE PEPPERS AND CAYENNE

Serves: 4

Prep time:
20 minutes

Cook time:
25 minutes

Level: Easy

Budget: $$

The peppers adorning this fish add a beautiful earthy color and a kick of fire. Choosing cod protects you from mercury and other toxins usually found in larger predatory fish such as swordfish or tilefish.

- 1 tablespoon plus 1 teaspoon extra-virgin olive oil
- 1 medium poblano pepper
- ½ jalapeño pepper
- 1 garlic clove
- ½ shallot, chopped
- ¼ teaspoon cayenne pepper
- ½ teaspoon sea salt
- 4 (6-ounce) skinless cod fillets

1. Preheat the oven to 350°F. Grease a baking sheet with 1 teaspoon of the oil and set aside.
2. Rub the peppers with ½ teaspoon of the oil and roast them over an open flame, on a grill, or in the oven under the broiler element until the skin is completely charred. Place the peppers in a bowl and cover tightly with plastic wrap. Let sit for 5 minutes, peel away all blackened skin, and remove the seeds and stems.
3. Combine the roasted peppers, remaining 2½ teaspoons olive oil, garlic, shallot, cayenne, and salt in a food processor and purée until completely smooth.
4. Place the cod on the baking sheet and spread the puréed roasted pepper mixture evenly over the fish.
5. Bake until the fish flakes easily when tested with a fork, 20–25 minutes.
6. Transfer to a platter and serve. Leftover fish can be refrigerated overnight but is best when served the same day.

Nutritional analysis per serving (1 fillet): calories 234, fat 6 g, saturated fat 1 g, cholesterol 98 mg, fiber 0 g, protein 41 g, carbohydrate 2 g, sodium 251 mg

WASABI SALMON SALAD

Wasabi is a Japanese condiment classically served with sushi. It is a spicy horse-radish, and the flavor dissolves rapidly in the mouth. Its addition gives this recipe a wonderful, though not overwhelming, spicy flavor.

- 1 (6-ounce) can wild salmon, drained
- 2 scallions, minced
- 1 celery rib, finely chopped
- ½-inch piece fresh ginger, peeled and grated
- ½ cup plain, unsweetened soy yogurt
- ¼ teaspoon wasabi paste
- sea salt and freshly ground black pepper
- 2 cups chopped Napa cabbage or bok choy

1. In a medium bowl, combine the salmon, scallions, celery, grated ginger, soy yogurt, and wasabi and toss gently until well mixed.
2. Season the mixture to taste with salt and black pepper and serve over a bed of Napa cabbage or bok choy. Any leftover salad can be refrigerated for up to 3 days.

Nutritional analysis per serving (½ cup salmon salad, 1 cup cabbage): calories 216, fat 8 g, saturated fat 2 g, cholesterol 37 mg, fiber 2 g, protein 21 g, carbohydrate 15 g, sodium 370 mg

Serves: 2

Prep time: 15 minutes

Level: Easy

Budget: $

SPICY SALMON SALAD

Serves: 3

Prep time:
10 minutes

Level: Easy

Budget: $

Simple, quick lunches are easy if you have the ingredients on hand. Combining different flavors and spices like jalapeños, cilantro, garlic, and cayenne spices up omega-3-rich salmon. Consider adding garbanzo beans to add even more fiber and protein to this meal.

DRESSING:

- juice of ½ lime
- 2 tablespoons balsamic vinegar
- 1 garlic clove, minced
- 1 teaspoon ground cumin
- 1 teaspoon chili powder
- ⅛ teaspoon cayenne pepper
- sea salt and freshly ground black pepper
- 2 tablespoons extra-virgin olive oil

SALAD:

- 1 (14-ounce) can wild salmon, drained
- 3 scallions, finely chopped
- ½ red bell pepper, seeded and chopped
- ½ jalapeño pepper, seeded and finely chopped
- ½ cup chopped fresh cilantro
- 6 kalamata olives, pitted and thinly sliced

MAKE THE DRESSING:

In a small bowl whisk together the lime juice, balsamic vinegar, garlic, cumin, chili powder, cayenne, and salt and pepper to taste. While whisking, slowly drizzle in the olive oil until it thickens slightly and emulsifies. Taste for seasoning and add more salt or black pepper if needed.

ASSEMBLE THE SALAD:

1. In a medium bowl combine the salmon, scallions, bell pepper, jalapeño, cilantro, and olives and toss until mixed well.

2. Pour half of the dressing over the salmon and vegetables and toss lightly. Add more dressing to taste. Any leftovers can be stored in the refrigerator for up to 2 days.

Nutritional analysis per serving (1 cup): calories 242, fat 16 g, saturated fat 3 g, cholesterol 36 mg, fiber 5 g, protein 2 g, carbohydrate 23 g, sodium 203 mg

BAKED SALMON CAKES

Serves: 2

Prep time:
5 minutes

Cook time:
30 minutes

Level: Easy

Budget: $

A simple, delicious, protein- and omega-3-rich addition to any meal.

- 1 tablespoon grapeseed oil
- 6 ounces cooked salmon or 1 (6-ounce) can wild salmon, undrained
- ½ medium red onion, finely chopped
- 1 large egg, beaten
- ¼ cup finely chopped almonds
- ½ teaspoon sea salt
- ¼ teaspoon freshly ground black pepper
- 1 cup almond meal, or more if needed
- 1 lemon, cut into wedges

1. Preheat the oven to 425°F. Lightly grease a baking sheet with the oil and put it in the oven on the top rack to preheat.

2. In a medium bowl, shred the salmon into small flakes with two forks. (If using canned salmon, pour the liquid from the can into the bowl, too.)

3. Add the onion, egg, almonds, salt, and pepper and mix well.

4. Stir in the almond meal. Test the mixture to see if it holds its shape when formed: take a small handful of salmon and try to form it into a small patty. If it holds its shape and doesn't seem to be falling apart, don't add any more almond meal. If it is still loose and mushy, add a couple more tablespoons of almond meal, mix, and test again. Once you are able to shape the salmon cakes, form two large, equal patties.

5. Season both sides of the cakes to taste with salt and black pepper and put them on the preheated baking sheet. Slide the tray back into the oven and bake on the top rack for 20 minutes, turning the cakes once after the first 10 minutes of cooking.

6. Remove the salmon cakes from the oven when they are golden brown and slightly crisp on both sides. Let them cool for 5 minutes on a wire rack before serving. Serve with the lemon wedges.

Nutritional analysis per serving (1 cake): calories 432, fat 31 g, saturated fat 4 g, cholesterol 93 mg, fiber 5 g, protein 23 g, carbohydrate 12 g, sodium 107 mg

Almond-Crusted Salmon with Lentil Salad

Serves: 2

Prep time:
15 minutes

Cook time:
10 minutes

Level: Easy

Budget: $

This crispy, crusty salmon, rich with the nutty flavor of lentils, is full of protein, fiber, nutrients, and minerals—many important things missing from our diet. The lemon zest makes it especially refreshing. Sumac, typical in Middle Eastern cuisine, is used to add freshness and lemon essence. Great on hummus!

SALMON:

- ½ cup toasted unsalted almonds
- zest of 1 lemon
- 2 tablespoon chopped fresh parsley
- 2 (6-ounce) skin-on wild salmon fillets
- 1 teaspoon sea salt
- ½ teaspoon freshly ground black pepper
- 2 tablespoons grapeseed oil

DRESSING:

- 1 tablespoon lemon juice
- 1 tablespoon apple cider vinegar
- 1 tablespoon chopped fresh parsley
- ½ teaspoon sumac
- 2 tablespoons extra-virgin olive oil
- sea salt and freshly ground black pepper

SALAD:

- 1 cup cooked lentils
- 1 large cucumber, chopped
- 1 large tomato, chopped
- 1 avocado, peeled, pitted, and chopped

MAKE THE SALMON:

1. Combine the almonds, lemon zest, and parsley in a food processor and pulse until finely ground. You want the mixture to be as fine as fresh breadcrumbs. Spread it out on a large plate.

2. Remove any pin bones from the salmon fillets and pat them dry with a paper towel. Season both sides of the fillets with the salt and black pepper.

3. Put the salmon fillets, flesh side down, on the plate of ground almonds. (You do not want to crust the skin side.) Press the salmon into the almond mixture. Transfer to a clean plate, skin side down.

4. Heat the grapeseed oil in a large cast-iron pan or sauté pan over medium-high heat. Once the oil is very hot, carefully place the fillets skin-side down in the pan. Cook without disturbing the fillets until the skin is crispy and golden brown and it releases from the pan easily, about 6 minutes.

5. Carefully turn over the fillets with two spatulas and cook until the almond crust is golden brown and the fish is as done as you like, 3–4 minutes. Let the fish rest for 3 minutes before serving.

MAKE THE DRESSING:

While the salmon is resting, combine the lemon juice, apple cider vinegar, parsley, and sumac in a blender. Turn the blender on medium speed, slowly drizzle in the oil, and season to taste with salt and black pepper. Blend for 1 minute.

ASSEMBLE THE SALAD:

1. Combine all of the salad ingredients in a bowl, pour in half of the dressing, and gently toss the salad. Taste and add more dressing as desired.

2. Lay half of the salad out onto each plate to form a bed and place a warm salmon fillet on top. Serve immediately.

Nutritional analysis per serving (1 fillet, 1 cup salad): calories 520, fat 28 g, saturated fat 4 g, cholesterol 61 mg, fiber 13 g, protein 33 g, carbohydrate 28 g, sodium 643 mg

Slow-Baked Salmon

Serves: 2

Prep time:
5 minutes

Cook time:
15 minutes

Level: Easy

Budget: $$

Salmon is a favorite of mine because it is high in orange carotenoids (from the salmon eating the algae at the bottom of the sea) and rich in omega-3 fats— both have anti-inflammatory properties and antioxidants. This is an easily digested, blood-sugar-balancing, delicious source of protein.

- 1½ teaspoons extra-virgin olive oil
- 1 teaspoon chopped fresh thyme
- 1 lemon, zested and cut into wedges
- 1 (8-ounce) skin-on wild salmon fillet
- ¼ teaspoon sea salt
- ¼ teaspoon freshly ground black pepper

1. Preheat the oven to 275°F. Lightly grease a small baking sheet with ½ teaspoon of the oil and set aside.
2. In a small bowl combine the thyme, lemon zest, and the remaining 1 teaspoon oil, and whisk until well mixed.
3. Remove any pin bones from the salmon and pat it dry with a paper towel. Season both sides of the fillet with the salt and black pepper. Spread the thyme-oil mixture on both sides of the fillet and transfer it, skin side down, to the greased baking sheet.
4. Cook the fillet until the center is just opaque, about 15 minutes. Serve with the lemon wedges.

Nutritional analysis per serving (½ fillet): calories 205, fat 10 g, saturated fat 3 g, cholesterol 70 mg, fiber 1 g, protein 51 g, carbohydrate 2 g, sodium 56 mg

LEMON-DILL WILD SALMON

This flaky, moist fish is an excellent source of omega-3 fatty acids, which turn down inflammation and increase vitality.

Serves: 4

Prep time: 5 minutes

Cook time: 20 minutes

Level: Easy

Budget: $

- 1 tablespoon extra-virgin olive oil
- 3 garlic cloves, minced
- juice of 1 small lemon
- ½ teaspoon minced fresh dill
- ½ teaspoon minced fresh parsley
- ½ teaspoon minced fresh tarragon
- ½ teaspoon sea salt
- ¼ teaspoon freshly ground black pepper
- 4 (4-ounce) skin-on wild salmon fillets

1. Preheat the oven to 350°F. Grease a baking sheet with 1 teaspoon of the oil and set aside.

2. Combine the garlic, remaining 2 teaspoons olive oil, lemon juice, herbs, salt, and pepper in a bowl and stir until well mixed.

3. Place the salmon fillets, skin side down, on the baking sheet and evenly spread the herb mixture over the tops. Bake until the fish flakes easily when tested with a fork, 15–20 minutes.

4. Transfer to a platter and serve. Leftover salmon can be refrigerated overnight but is best when served the same day.

Nutritional analysis per serving (1 fillet): calories 196, fat 11 g, saturated fat 2 g, cholesterol 62 mg, fiber 0 g, protein 23 g, carbohydrate 1 g, sodium 52 mg

GRILLED WILD SALMON WITH MUSTARD-MINT SAUCE AND STEAMED BROCCOLI

Serves: 4

Prep time: 20 minutes

Cook time: 10 minutes

Chill time: 20

Level: Easy

Budget: $

Mustard and mint are classic flavors to serve with salmon. The result is a fresh, tangy, healthful dish loaded with omega-3 fats.

- ¼ cup fresh mint leaves
- 3 tablespoons Dijon mustard
- 2 tablespoons plus 2 teaspoons extra-virgin olive oil
- juice of ½ lemon
- 4 (4–ounce) wild salmon fillets, about 1 inch thick
- sea salt and freshly ground black pepper
- florets from 1 medium head broccoli, steamed

1. Preheat the grill. (If you don't have access to a grill, use the broiler element in your oven.)
2. Combine the mint, mustard, 2 tablespoons of the olive oil, and the lemon juice in a small food processor or blender and purée until smooth. Refrigerate for 15–20 minutes so the flavors will meld.
3. Run the salmon fillets under cold running water and pat them dry. Rub the salmon with the remaining 2 teaspoons olive oil and season to taste with salt and black pepper.
4. Lightly oil the grill grates and grill the salmon until it reaches the desired doneness (about 3 minutes per side for medium-rare).
5. Serve the salmon with the mustard–mint sauce and the steamed broccoli.

Nutritional analysis per serving (1 fillet, ¾ cup broccoli): calories 310, fat 14 g, saturated fat 3 g, cholesterol 65 mg, fiber 3 g, protein 33 g, carbohydrate 8 g, sodium 256 mg

CHILE VERDE CHICKEN

Serves: 4

Prep time: 15 minutes

Cook time: 30 minutes

Level: Easy

Budget: $

Spices are a wonderful way to enhance your diet with extra phytochemicals and antioxidants. Ingredients such as cilantro, jalapeños, cumin, and peppercorns have very powerful medicinal effects on your body. And the good news is that they make your chicken taste fabulous!

VERDE SAUCE:

- 3 cups low-sodium chicken broth
- 16 small tomatillos, husked
- 2 jalapeño peppers, seeded and halved
- 3 garlic cloves, peeled
- 1 large white onion, chopped
- 1 bunch cilantro (about 3 ounces)
- 1 teaspoon ground cumin
- juice of 2 limes
- sea salt and freshly ground black pepper to taste

CHICKEN:

- 2 tablespoons extra-virgin olive oil
- sea salt and freshly ground black pepper
- 4 (5-ounce) boneless, skinless chicken breasts

MAKE THE VERDE SAUCE:

1. Heat the broth in a medium pot over high heat. Once it boils, reduce the heat to medium–low and add the tomatillos, jalapeños, and garlic cloves. Cook at a brisk simmer until the vegetables are soft, 5–6 minutes.

2. Transfer the contents of the pot to a blender. Add the onion, cilantro, cumin, lime juice, salt, and black pepper while the blender is running. Blend until smooth, about 2 minutes. Set aside.

MAKE THE CHICKEN:

1. Heat the oil in a large sauté pan over medium-high heat. Season the chicken breasts generously with salt and black pepper and add them to

223

the hot pan. Cook until all the chicken pieces are brown, about 3 minutes per side.

2. Reduce the heat to low and add the blended verde sauce. Cover the pan and simmer until the chicken is very tender, 20–25 minutes.

3. Shred the chicken with two forks and serve in the verde sauce. Any leftover chicken can be refrigerated for up to 3 days.

Nutritional analysis per serving (1½ cups shredded chicken and sauce): calories 272, fat 11 g, saturated fat 2 g, cholesterol 73 mg, fiber 3 g, protein 30 g, carbohydrate 12 g, sodium 188 mg

ALMOND-FLAX-CRUSTED CHICKEN

Serves: 4

Prep time: 10 minutes

Cook time: 30 minutes

Level: Easy

Budget: $

The nutty crust enveloping this chicken ensures it will be moist and tender. Using almond meal lowers the glycemic load and adds flavor, fiber, and protein to satisfy you with each mouth-watering bite.

- 4 (5-ounce) boneless, skinless chicken breasts
- 3 tablespoons ground flaxseeds
- ½ cup almond meal
- 1 tablespoon plus 1 teaspoon extra-virgin olive oil
- 1 tablespoon almond butter
- 1 tablespoon finely chopped yellow onion
- 1 teaspoon lemon juice
- 1 teaspoon sea salt
- pinch of cayenne pepper
- ¼ teaspoon paprika
- 1 teaspoon chopped fresh parsley
- 1 teaspoon chopped fresh thyme

1. Preheat the oven to 350°F. Oil a baking sheet with 1 teaspoon oil and set it aside.

2. Place the chicken breasts between two sheets of plastic wrap or parchment paper and pound them with a kitchen mallet until the pieces are approximately ½ inch thick.

3. Pour the flax and almond meal into a small bowl and stir until evenly mixed.

4. In another small bowl, combine all of the remaining ingredients. Add the chicken breasts to this mixture and toss them until coated. (If time allows, marinate the chicken in the mixture for 10–15 minutes to further enhance flavor.)

5. Remove the chicken pieces from the marinade and transfer them to the baking sheet. Sprinkle half of the almond/flax crust over the tops of the chicken breasts and gently press the crust into each piece until

evenly coated. Carefully turn the chicken over and repeat the process with the remaining almond/flax mixture.

6. Put the baking sheet into the oven on the top rack and bake until the juices run clear, 20–30 minutes. Any leftover chicken can be refrigerated for up to 3 days.

Nutritional analysis per serving (1 breast): calories 349, fat 18 g, saturated fat 2 g, cholesterol 82 mg, fiber 6 g, protein 40 g, carbohydrate 8 g, sodium 197 mg

CURRIED COCONUT CHICKEN BREASTS

The fat from coconuts is very healthy and carries the flavors and aromas of the curry.

- 2 teaspoons extra-virgin olive oil
- ½-inch piece fresh ginger, peeled and minced
- 1 garlic clove, minced
- 3 scallions (green parts only), minced
- 1 teaspoon minced fresh parsley
- 2 teaspoons curry powder
- ½ teaspoon sea salt
- ⅛ teaspoon cayenne pepper
- 1 tablespoon unsweetened coconut milk
- 4 (5-ounce) boneless, skinless chicken breasts

Serves: 4

Prep time: 20 minutes

Cook time: 30 minutes

Level: Easy

Budget: $

1. Preheat the oven to 350°F. Lightly grease a baking sheet with the oil and set it aside.
2. Combine all of the ingredients except for the chicken in a bowl and mix well. Place the chicken breasts in the bowl and toss them in the marinade until evenly coated. Allow the chicken to sit for 10–15 minutes.
3. Remove the chicken breasts from the marinade and transfer them to the baking sheet. Place the baking sheet on the top rack in the oven and bake until the juices run clear, 20–30 minutes. Any leftover chicken can be refrigerated for up to 3 days.

Nutritional analysis per serving (1 breast): calories 189, fat 5 g, saturated fat 2 g, cholesterol 82 mg, fiber 0 g, protein 33 g, carbohydrate 1 g, sodium 221 mg

GRILLED ROSEMARY CHICKEN BREASTS

Serves: 4

Prep time:
15 minutes

Cook time:
15 minutes

Level: Easy

Budget: $

Rosemary is slightly lemony and invigorating, especially when its oils are released with the heat from the grill. Use an indoor grill pan seasoned with olive oil if you don't want to go outdoors.

- 1 garlic clove, peeled
- 1 tablespoon extra-virgin olive oil
- ⅛ teaspoon cayenne pepper
- 2 teaspoons chopped fresh rosemary
- 1 teaspoon chopped fresh parsley
- ½ teaspoon sea salt
- 4 (5-ounce) boneless, skinless chicken breasts

1. Preheat the grill.
2. Combine the garlic, oil, cayenne pepper, herbs, and salt in a small food processor and pulse until the garlic is finely chopped.
3. Place the chicken breasts a medium bowl and add the garlic herb mixture. Toss the chicken until it is evenly coated and let it marinate for 10–15 minutes before grilling.
4. Lightly oil the grill grates and grill the chicken for 10–12 minutes, turning once halfway through the cooking. The chicken is done when it is firm to the touch and lightly charred on both sides. Serve immediately. Any leftover chicken can be refrigerated for up to 3 days.

Nutritional analysis per serving (1 breast): calories 188, fat 5 g, saturated fat 1 g, cholesterol 82 mg, fiber 0 g, protein 33 g, carbohydrate 0 g, sodium 220 mg

LEMON-GARLIC-BASIL CHICKEN

The basil tastes amazingly fresh and has a distinct aroma sure to please every palate. This meal is quick to prepare but will stay with you for hours thanks to the lean protein from the chicken.

- 2 teaspoons extra-virgin olive oil
- 1 garlic clove, peeled
- ¼ teaspoon cayenne pepper
- juice of ½ small lemon
- 3 teaspoons chopped fresh basil
- ½ teaspoon sea salt
- 4 (5-ounce) boneless, skinless chicken breasts

Serves: 4

Prep time: 15 minutes

Cook time: 30 minutes

Level: Easy

Budget: $

1. Preheat the oven to 350°F. Lightly grease a baking sheet with ½ teaspoon of the oil and set aside.
2. Combine the garlic, cayenne pepper, lemon juice, basil, salt, and remaining 1½ teaspoons oil in a small food processor and pulse until the garlic is finely chopped.
3. Place the chicken breasts in a medium bowl and add the garlic-basil mixture. Toss the chicken until evenly coated and let it marinate for 10–15 minutes.
4. Transfer the chicken breasts to the baking sheet and put the baking sheet in the oven on the top rack. Bake the chicken for 20–30 minutes, turning once halfway through the cooking. The chicken is done when it's firm to the touch and the juices run clear. Any leftover chicken can be refrigerated for up to 3 days.

Nutritional analysis per serving (1 breast): calories 187, fat 4 g, saturated fat 1 g, cholesterol 82 mg, fiber 0 g, protein 33 g, carbohydrate 3 g, sodium 228 mg

ROAST TURKEY BREAST AND AVOCADO CREAM ON A BED OF GREENS

Serves: 2

Prep time:
20 minutes

Level: Easy

Budget: $

The light, refreshing dressing for this dish contains avocados, a healthy source of monounsaturated fats. The dressing keeps well in the fridge, so make it up to 3 days ahead of time and enjoy with turkey, chicken, or fish.

AVOCADO CREAM:

- 1 avocado, peeled and pitted
- juice of 1 large lemon
- 3 tablespoons extra-virgin olive oil
- 1 garlic clove, peeled
- sea salt and freshly ground black pepper to taste
- 3–4 tablespoons water

SALAD:

- 6 cups mixed baby greens
- 6 ounces roasted turkey breast, sliced
- ½ small red onion, thinly sliced
- 1 pickling cucumber, thinly sliced
- 10 green olives, pitted and chopped

MAKE THE AVOCADO CREAM:

1. Place the avocado, lemon juice, olive oil, garlic, salt, and black pepper in a food processor and process until very smooth, 1–2 minutes.
2. Slowly add the water and continue processing until the dressing is thick and creamy.

ASSEMBLE THE SALAD:

Divide the greens between two serving plates. Top with the sliced turkey, red onion, cucumber, and green olives. Drizzle over the avocado dressing and serve. Stored separately, the turkey salad and dressing will keep for 3 days in the refrigerator.

Nutritional analysis per serving (3 ounces turkey, ½ cup avocado cream, about 3½ cups salad): calories 494, fat 38 g, saturated fat 5 g, cholesterol 46 mg, fiber 9 g, protein 25 g, carbohydrate 19 g, sodium 526 mg

Spiced Ground Turkey Wrap with Watercress and Avocado

Serves: 1

Prep time: 10 minutes

Cook time: 20 minutes

Level: Easy

Budget: $

I held a recipe contest and this recipe won in the Advanced Plan category. My son and his friends love this easy-to-make treat. It's tangy, tasty, and unusual—spicy turkey with crisp watercress, creamy avocado, and crunchy romaine leaves.

SPICED TURKEY:

- 2 tablespoons extra-virgin olive oil
- ½ medium yellow onion, thinly sliced
- 2 garlic cloves, minced
- 1-inch piece fresh ginger, peeled and minced
- 1 medium carrot, peeled and shredded
- ¼ teaspoon cayenne pepper
- ¼ teaspoon ground coriander
- ¼ teaspoon ground turmeric
- ⅛ teaspoon ground cinnamon
- ¼ teaspoon sea salt
- ¼ teaspoon freshly ground black pepper
- 5 ounces lean ground turkey
- 2 tablespoons low-sodium chicken broth
- 1 tablespoon finely chopped fresh cilantro

WRAPS:

- 4 large romaine leaves
- ½ avocado, peeled, pitted, and mashed
- ½ cup baby spinach
- ½ cup watercress
- 1 lime, cut into wedges

MAKE THE TURKEY:

1. Heat the oil in a wok or large cast-iron pan over medium-high heat. Sauté the onion, garlic, and ginger, stirring constantly, until aromatic and softened, 3–4 minutes.

2. Add the carrot, cayenne, coriander, turmeric, and cinnamon. Season to taste with salt and black pepper and mix well. After a minute add the turkey, breaking it up with a spoon. Cook the turkey, stirring frequently, until browned, 6–8 minutes.

3. Pour in the chicken broth and stir, scraping the bottom of the pan to release any tasty browned bits. Turn off the heat and fold in the cilantro. Transfer the turkey mixture to a small bowl.

ASSEMBLE THE WRAPS:

Lay the lettuce leaves out on a plate and spread a heaping teaspoon of the mashed avocado on each leaf. Add some spinach and watercress to each wrap. Top with small piles of the spiced turkey and roll up. Serve with the lime wedges on the side.

Nutritional analysis per serving (4 wraps): calories 566, fat 36 g, saturated fat 5 g, cholesterol 70 mg, fiber 9 g, protein 40 g, carbohydrate 27 g, sodium 314 mg

Apricot-Glazed Pork and Vegetable Stir-Fry over Sautéed Greens

Serves: 4

Prep time: 30 minutes

Cook time: 15 minutes

Level: Easy

Budget: $

The sauce for this dish is a bit like a Thai peanut sauce; however, the addition of apricot, mustard, and rice vinegar offers sweetness and tang you don't get in a traditional peanut sauce. It's delicious on pork, but you can use it on chicken and other light meats as well.

- 2 tablespoons rice vinegar
- 3 tablespoons chunky peanut butter
- 1 tablespoon Dijon mustard
- ½ teaspoon ground allspice
- 4 fresh apricots, peeled, pitted, and finely chopped
- 2 tablespoons sesame seeds
- ½-inch piece fresh ginger, peeled and grated
- 2 garlic cloves, minced
- ½ teaspoon sea salt
- 1¼ pounds pork tenderloin, cut into 1-inch-thick medallions
- 1 tablespoon plus 1 teaspoon extra-virgin coconut oil
- 1 large carrot, peeled and thinly sliced
- ½ large head broccoli, cut into medium florets
- 1 red bell pepper, seeded and thinly sliced
- 1 cup shiitake mushrooms, stemmed and thickly sliced
- 4 cups chopped bok choy
- 2 scallions, thinly sliced
- 1 tablespoon olive oil
- 2 cups mixed greens (such as kale, Swiss chard, or mustard greens)

1. Whisk the rice vinegar, peanut butter, Dijon mustard, and allspice together in a small saucepan until smooth. Add the apricots to the pan and turn the heat to medium. Once simmering, cook the sauce until it thickens, 3–5 minutes. Remove from the heat and set aside.

2. In a large bowl, combine the sesame seeds, ginger, garlic, and salt. Add the pork and toss until all of the medallions are evenly coated.

3. Heat a wok or large cast-iron pan over medium-high heat and add the coconut oil. After a minute carefully add the pork and cook, turning once halfway, until cooked through, 3–4 minutes per side.

4. Remove the pork and transfer it to a plate to rest. Add the carrot, broccoli, red pepper, mushrooms, bok choy, and scallions. Stir-fry until the vegetables are tender but still crisp, 4–5 minutes.

5. To sauté the greens, heat a sauté pan over medium-high to high heat. Coat the pan with about 1 tablespoon olive oil. Add the greens and stir over medium heat until the leaves begin to wilt, 2–3 minutes. Remove from the heat.

6. Return the pork to the wok, along with any juices that might have accumulated on the plate, and pour the apricot glaze over the pork and vegetables. Stir-fry until the sauce reduces and all the pork pieces are nicely glazed, 3–4 minutes. Serve over the sautéed greens. Any leftover pork and vegetables can be refrigerated for up to 3 days.

Nutritional analysis per serving (2 medallions): calories 414, fat 18 g, saturated fat 3 g, cholesterol 92 mg, fiber 7 g, protein 38 g, carbohydrate 29 g, sodium 174 mg

Serves: 2

Prep time:
5 minutes

Chill time:
30 minutes

Level: Easy

Budget: $

SNACKS AND SIDES

MATCHA GREEN ENERGIZER

This powerful healing cocktail may sound unusual, but I urge you to try it. Matcha green tea is made from whole tea leaves; but rather than overstimulating you like coffee, it provides relaxed mental alertness, while detoxifying and alkalizing your blood and regulating your blood sugar. It contains high levels of antioxidants, even more than blueberries. L-theanine, an amino acid that calms the brain, is abundant in matcha leaves. It helps to lower stress levels, lower blood pressure, and even improve memory. Aloe vera is a great cleansing and detoxifying plant with antimicrobial activity. In appropriate doses, aloe vera juice can be used as a tonic and anti-inflammatory agent to help everything from osteoarthritis to colitis. Ginger juice is a medicinal extract from the ginger plant that offers spice and warmth. If you are looking for a quick pick-me-up, this is it.

- 1 large celery rib
- 1 medium apple
- 1 cup baby spinach
- 1 large kale leaf
- 1 large cucumber
- 2 tablespoons aloe vera juice
- juice of 1 lime
- ¼ cup ginger juice
- 2 teaspoons matcha green tea powder

1. Using an electric juicer, juice the celery, apple, spinach, kale, and cucumber into a measuring cup or small pitcher. (If you don't have a juicer, you can prepare this in a blender—peel the cucumber, peel and core the apple, and stem the kale before blending. Add a splash of water to help the blender get started.)

2. Add the aloe vera juice, lime juice, and ginger juice, and stir in the matcha green tea powder. Refrigerate for 30 minutes and serve chilled.

Nutritional analysis per serving (¾ cup): calories 73, fat 0.3 g, saturated fat 0 g, cholesterol 0 mg, fiber 4 g, protein 2 g, carbohydrate 19 g, sodium 33 mg

TUSCAN BEANS

This is one of my favorite quick and easy snacks—it's a staple in my home and I'm sure it'll become one of your family favorites in no time.

- 2 tablespoons extra-virgin olive oil
- ½ tablespoon finely chopped fresh rosemary
- 1 medium yellow onion, chopped
- 2 cups cooked cannellini beans or 1 (15-ounce) can cannellini beans, rinsed and drained
- sea salt

1. Heat the oil in a medium saucepan over medium heat. Add the rosemary and onions and sauté until the onions soften slightly, about 3 minutes.

2. Pour in the beans and season them to taste with salt. Stir the mixture until evenly mixed and cook until the beans are just warmed through. Remove the pan from the heat and transfer the beans to a serving dish. Serve warm or at room temperature. Any leftover beans can be refrigerated for up to 4 days.

Nutritional analysis per serving (½ cup): calories 143, fat 8 g, saturated fat 1 g, cholesterol 0 mg, fiber 4 g, protein 5 g, carbohydrate 15 g, sodium 142 mg

Serves: 4

Prep time: 5 minutes

Cook time: 5 minutes

Level: Easy

Budget: $

DELUXE GUACAMOLE

Serves: 4

Prep time:
5 minutes

Level: Easy

Budget: $

This guacamole is rich in fiber, protein, and good fats and is combined with delicious flavors like cilantro, cumin, and cayenne. Dip celery, carrots, or lettuce leaves into the guacamole instead of tortilla chips.

- 2 avocados, halved, pits reserved
- 3 garlic cloves, minced
- ½ medium white onion, finely chopped
- ¼ cup chopped fresh cilantro, a few leaves reserved for garnish
- 2 teaspoons ground cumin
- ⅛ teaspoon cayenne pepper
- juice of 1 lime
- sea salt to taste
- 1 medium tomato, finely chopped

1. Scoop out the avocado flesh with a large spoon and place in a medium bowl. Using a large fork or potato masher, mash the avocados until spreadable but still chunky.

2. Add the garlic, onion, cilantro, cumin, cayenne pepper, lime juice, and salt and stir to combine. Taste for seasoning and adjust with more salt or lime juice if needed.

3. Garnish with the tomato and a few cilantro leaves. Serve with celery, carrots, or lettuce leaves. Any leftover guacamole can be stored in the refrigerator for up to 3 days. (To help prevent browning, place an avocado pit in the mixture and put a layer of plastic wrap on the surface of the dip before covering the container.)

Nutritional analysis per serving (½ cup): calories 178, fat 16 g, saturated fat 1 g, cholesterol 0 mg, fiber 8 g, protein 3 g, carbohydrate 15 g, sodium 306 mg

LISA'S FAMOUS GUACAMOLE

Here is another fabulous guacamole recipe with fresh jalapeños to give it a little extra heat and an anti-inflammatory kick.

- 5 avocados, halved, pits reserved
- 2 garlic cloves, minced
- 1 medium red onion, finely chopped
- ½ cup chopped fresh cilantro, a few leaves reserved for garnish
- 1 jalapeño pepper, seeded and finely chopped
- juice of 2 limes
- sea salt to taste
- 1 medium tomato, finely chopped

Serves: 10

Prep time: 10 minutes

Level: Easy

Budget: $

1. Scoop out the avocado flesh with a large spoon and place in a medium bowl. Using a large fork or potato masher, mash the avocados until spreadable but still chunky.

2. Add the garlic, onion, cilantro, jalapeño, lime juice, and salt and stir to combine. Taste for seasoning and adjust with additional salt or lime juice if needed.

3. Garnish with the tomato and a few cilantro leaves. Serve with raw crunchy vegetables such as celery, sugar snap peas, carrots, jicama, etc. Any leftover guacamole can be stored in the refrigerator for up to 3 days. (To help prevent browning, place an avocado pit in the mixture and put a layer of plastic wrap on the surface of the dip before covering the container.)

Nutritional analysis per serving (⅓ cup): calories 102, fat 9 g, saturated fat 1 g, cholesterol 0 mg, fiber 4 g, protein 1 g, carbohydrate 6 g, sodium 130 mg

GUACO TACOS

Serves: 6

Prep time:
15 minutes

Level: Easy

Budget: $

You can have your tacos and eat them, too, with this wonderfully creative recipe using sliced jicama, a crunchy, low-glycemic vegetable, as your taco shell. Filled with delicious guacamole, you will have the wonderful crunch of a taco and none of the blood sugar effects.

- 2 avocados, halved, pits reserved
- ½ small red onion, finely chopped
- ½ cup chopped fresh cilantro, a few leaves reserved for garnish
- 1 jalapeño pepper, seeded and finely chopped
- juice of 2 limes
- juice of ½ orange
- ¼ teaspoon sea salt
- 1 large jicama, peeled
- 1 lime, cut into wedges

1. Scoop out the avocado flesh with a large spoon and place in a medium bowl. Using a large fork or potato masher, mash the avocados until spreadable but still chunky.

2. Add the onion, cilantro, jalapeño, lime juice, orange juice, and salt and stir to combine. Taste for seasoning and adjust with more salt or lime juice if needed.

3. Using a mandolin or very sharp knife, slice the jicama into six ⅛-inch-thick rounds at the widest part of the jicama, close to the center, so you're left with the largest possible circular slices. These will be the "tortillas" for your tacos.

4. Lay the jicama "tortillas" flat and fill each with a couple of tablespoons of guacamole. Fold together like a taco and serve garnished with a few cilantro leaves and some lime wedges. Leftover guacamole can be stored in the refrigerator for up to 3 days. (To help prevent browning, place an avocado pit in the mixture and put a layer

of plastic wrap on the surface of the dip before covering the container.)

Nutritional analysis per serving (1 taco): calories 169, fat 10 g, saturated fat 1 g, cholesterol 0 mg, fiber 11 g, protein 3 g, carbohydrate 21 g, sodium 167 mg

Herbed Tomato Spread

Serves: 4

Prep time: 15 minutes

Level: Easy

Budget: $

Traditionally used as a topping on grilled bread in the wonderful Italian appetizer bruschetta, this tomato mixture can be eaten as a dip for vegetables or used as a condiment for chicken or fish.

- 5 medium tomatoes, finely chopped
- 4 garlic cloves, minced
- ¼ cup finely chopped fresh basil
- 3 tablespoons white balsamic vinegar
- 3 tablespoons extra-virgin olive oil
- sea salt and freshly ground black pepper to taste

1. Combine all of the ingredients in a medium bowl and stir until well mixed. Check for seasoning and add more salt and black pepper if needed.

2. Serve as a dip or alongside your protein of choice. The tomato spread is best if eaten the same day.

Nutritional analysis per serving (½ cup): calories 103, fat 57 g, saturated fat 1 g, cholesterol 0 mg, fiber 2 g, protein 2 g, carbohydrate 9 g, sodium 21 mg

CRISPY KALE CHIPS WITH SEA SALT

An indulgent side dish for dinner—or a healthier snack alternative to chips. Roasting brings out smoky, buttery flavors and creates an irresistible, melt-in-your-mouth texture. Roasting to the point of crispness at high heat does involve some nutritional sacrifices, but it's such a simple and delicious preparation (and one that has earned kale so many fans), it's worth making now and then. You can also cook the kale longer at a lower temperature, if you prefer. And if you're not afraid of fat, you can be more generous with the oil. For a twist, substitute Cajun spice or lemon pepper for the salt.

Serves: 2

Prep time: 5 minutes

Cook time: 15 minutes

Level: Easy

Budget: $

- 1 large bunch kale, stemmed and chopped into 3-inch pieces
- 1 tablespoon extra-virgin olive oil
- sea salt to taste

1. Preheat the oven to 375°F. Line a baking sheet with parchment paper.

2. Toss the kale pieces in a bowl with the olive oil until coated, then arrange in a single layer on the baking sheet.

3. Roast the kale for 5 minutes, then carefully turn the pieces over with metal tongs and roast until the kale begins turning brown, crisp, and brittle, 7–10 minutes. Remove from the oven and sprinkle with sea salt. Serve promptly or store in paper bags. If the chips lose their crunch, reheat them in a low oven until crisp, 3–4 minutes.

Nutritional analysis per serving (1 cup): calories 127, fat 8 g, saturated fat 1 g, cholesterol 0 mg, fiber 3 g, protein 5 g, carbohydrate 14 g, sodium 994 mg

Cashew "Cheese"

If you miss dairy cheese, try this recipe. It satisfies your cheesy, salty cravings and has wonderful fat, protein, and carbohydrates. It is good for your body and good for your soul. Probiotic powder adds healthy bacteria, which aids digestion, boosts immunity, and increases the nutrition availability in the gut; simply mix with filtered water to prepare. Nutritional yeast provides a "cheesy" flavor and is used to complement vegetarian dishes such as stews, grains, legumes, and veggies. It can be a source of vitamin B_{12} for vegetarians and vegans if it is properly fortified.

- 2 cups raw cashews, soaked overnight in water and drained
- 2 teaspoons probiotic powder
- ½ cup water
- 3 tablespoons finely chopped fresh basil
- 3 tablespoons finely chopped fresh parsley
- 3 tablespoons finely chopped fresh tarragon
- 2 teaspoons lemon juice
- 1 tablespoon plus 2 teaspoons nutritional yeast
- 1½ teaspoons sea salt
- ¼ teaspoon freshly ground black pepper

1. Put the cashews, probiotic powder, and water in a blender and blend on high speed until smooth, 2–3 minutes.
2. Transfer the blended cashew mixture to a glass bowl and cover with a kitchen towel. Leave the bowl on the kitchen counter for 12–24 hours.
3. Stir in the fresh herbs, lemon juice, nutritional yeast, salt, and black pepper.

4. Transfer the cheese to two 3-inch ramekins. Cover with plastic wrap and refrigerate for at least 12 hours before serving. Leftover cashew cheese can be refrigerated for up to 5 days.

Nutritional analysis per serving (about 2 tablespoons): calories 141, fat 11 g, saturated fat 2 g, cholesterol 0 mg, fiber 1 g, protein 4 g, carbohydrate 9 g, sodium 300 mg

OLIVE TAPENADE WITH RAW VEGETABLES

Serves: 6

Prep time:
5 minutes

Cook time:
20 minutes

Level: Easy

Budget: $

This slightly salty and savory snack will satisfy taste buds looking to complement fresh, crispy vegetables with something a little different. The roasted garlic deepens the flavor of this tapenade and also provides a boost to your immune system.

- 1 head garlic
- 1 tablespoon extra-virgin olive oil
- ½ cup kalamata olives, pitted
- ½ cup green olives, pitted
- juice of ½ lemon
- 4 cups mixed raw vegetables for dipping

1. Preheat the oven to 350°F.
2. Split the garlic head in half and brush it all over with the oil. Put the halves back together and wrap the garlic loosely in foil. Place the head of garlic on a baking sheet and roast for 20 minutes. When cool enough to handle, squeeze the roasted garlic cloves out of their skins into a food processor.
3. Add the olives and lemon juice to the food processor and puree until smooth. Any leftover tapenade can be refrigerated for up to 5 days.

Nutritional analysis per serving (1 tablespoon): calories 77, fat 5 g, saturated fat 0 g, cholesterol 7 mg, fiber 1 g, protein 1 g, carbohydrate 7 g, sodium 290 mg

ARTICHOKE DIP WITH RAW VEGGIES

Serves: 6

Prep time:
5 minutes

Chill time:
30 minutes

Level: Easy

Budget: $

Blended artichokes are the perfect way to indulge in a creamy and satisfying snack. They provide tons of blood-sugar-stabilizing fiber, magnesium, and potassium with little fat or calories. Enjoy with your favorite crunchy vegetables as a snack or at your next party.

- 1 (15-ounce) can artichoke hearts, drained
- 1 teaspoon extra-virgin olive oil
- 1 tablespoon dried Italian herb blend (or any combination of dried oregano, thyme, rosemary, and basil)
- sea salt to taste
- 4 cups mixed raw vegetables, for dipping

Place all of the ingredients except the raw vegetables in a food processor and blend until smooth, 30–60 seconds or until desired level of creaminess. Chill and serve the dip with the raw vegetables. Any leftover artichoke dip can be refrigerated for up to 5 days.

Nutritional analysis per serving (2 tablespoons): calories 27, fat 1 g, saturated fat 0 g, cholesterol 0 mg, fiber 2 g, protein 1 g, carbohydrate 4 g, sodium 230 mg

LEMONY HUMMUS WITH RAW VEGGIES

Serves: 10

Prep time:
20 minutes

Level: Easy

Budget: $

This hummus has a special lemony-garlicky essence that is absolutely wonderful as a dip for fresh vegetables. Finish it by drizzling a little extra-virgin olive oil over the top right before serving.

- 2 cups cooked chickpeas or 1 (15-ounce) can chickpeas, rinsed and drained
- ½ cup tahini
- 6 tablespoons extra-virgin olive oil
- juice of 2 small lemons
- 4 garlic cloves, peeled
- ½ teaspoon sea salt
- ¼ teaspoon freshly ground black pepper
- ⅛ teaspoon cayenne pepper
- 6 cups mixed raw vegetables, for dipping

1. Combine the chickpeas, tahini, 5 tablespoons of the olive oil, lemon juice, garlic, salt, black pepper, and cayenne pepper in a food processor. Blend until the mixture is smooth and creamy. If it is too thick, add 1–2 tablespoons water or more lemon juice until it reaches the consistency you desire.

2. Transfer to a bowl and drizzle with the remaining 1 tablespoon olive oil. Serve with the raw vegetables. Any leftover hummus can be refrigerated for up to 4 days.

Nutritional analysis per serving (2 tablespoons): calories 213, fat 17 g, saturated fat 2.2 g, cholesterol 0 mg, fiber 4 g, protein 5 g, carbohydrate 12 g, sodium 213 mg

GARLIC AND HERB HUMMUS

This hummus is best made ahead of time to allow the flavors to combine. For a tangier taste, use more lemon juice or add hot chili oil to spice it up.

- 3 garlic cloves, peeled
- 1 tablespoon extra-virgin olive oil
- 2 cups cooked chickpeas or 1 (15-ounce) can chickpeas, rinsed and drained
- ¼ cup tahini
- ½ cup water
- juice of ½ small lemon
- ½ teaspoon paprika
- 1 teaspoon chopped fresh parsley
- ¼ teaspoon cayenne pepper
- ¼ teaspoon sea salt

Serves: 4

Prep time: 5 minutes

Cook time: 25 minutes

Chill time: 20 minutes

Level: Easy

Budget: $

1. Preheat the oven to 350°F. Rub the garlic cloves with ½ teaspoon of the oil and wrap them loosely in foil. Place the garlic in the oven on the bottom rack and roast until soft, 20–25 minutes. Remove from the oven, open the foil, and let cool.

2. Combine the roasted garlic with the remaining ingredients in a food processor and blend the mixture into a fine paste.

3. Transfer the hummus to a bowl and serve. Any leftover hummus can be refrigerated for up to 4 days.

Nutritional analysis per serving (⅓ cup): calories 213, fat 17 g, saturated fat 2.2 g, cholesterol 0 mg, fiber 4 g, protein 5 g, carbohydrate 12 g, sodium 213 mg

SALMON PARTY PÂTÉ

Serves: 12

Prep time:
10 minutes

Chill time:
3 hours

Level: Easy

Budget: $$

Salmon pâté is a delicious and elegant spread for vegetables. Agar is made from seaweed and helps give the tofu-salmon mixture the right texture. It can be found at your local whole foods or natural foods market near the sea vegetables.

- 1 teaspoon agar
- 3 tablespoons hot water
- 1 pound firm tofu
- 6 ounces cooked, smoked, or drained canned salmon
- 2 tablespoons capers
- 1 tablespoon minced fresh dill
- juice of 1 lemon
- ¼ teaspoon cayenne pepper
- sea salt
- 1 small red onion, finely chopped
- 1 tablespoon capers
- 1 lemon, cut into wedges
- leaves from 2 large heads endive
- 6 celery ribs, halved

1. In a small bowl combine the agar and hot water. Let bloom for 5–10 minutes.
2. Combine the bloomed agar, tofu, salmon, capers, dill, lemon juice, and cayenne pepper in a food processor, season to taste with salt, and blend until smooth. Chill in the refrigerator until firm, 3–4 hours.
3. Serve the chilled pâté garnished with red onion, capers, and lemon wedges on a bed of endive leaves and celery sticks for dipping. The pâté can be wrapped tightly in plastic wrap and stored in the refrigerator for up to 2 days.

Nutritional analysis per serving (¹/₃ cup pâté): calories 101, fat 6 g, saturated fat 1 g, cholesterol 22 mg, fiber 0 g, protein 11 g, carbohydrate 1 g, sodium 147 mg

SHRIMP SALSA

A protein-rich salsa is a great addition to any meal. Try it with gluten-free seed crackers.

- 1 ½ pounds raw shrimp, peeled and deveined
- 1 large red onion, finely chopped
- 2 plum tomatoes, seeded and finely chopped
- 1 small jalapeño pepper, seeded and finely chopped
- 3 avocados, peeled, pitted, and finely chopped
- 1 large bunch cilantro (about 3 ounces), finely chopped
- 6 garlic cloves, finely chopped
- juice of 8 limes
- 1 (15-ounce) can tomato sauce
- sea salt and freshly ground black pepper
- 4 cups of sliced celery, cucumber, or other crunchy vegetables, for dipping

Serves: 8

Prep time: 10 minutes

Cook time: 5 minutes

Chill time: 3 hours

Level: Easy

Budget: $$

1. In a saucepan, bring about 2 quarts of water to a boil over high heat. Add the shrimp (add water if necessary so shrimp are covered with 1 inch of water) and cook until just pink, 2–3 minutes.

2. Drain the shrimp, reserving ¼ cup of the cooking liquid, and transfer the shrimp to a large bowl of ice water to stop them from cooking further. Once the shrimp are cold, drain and chop them into bite-size chunks.

3. Add the shrimp pieces to a large nonreactive container along with the onion, tomatoes, jalapeño, avocados, cilantro, garlic, lime juice, and tomato sauce. Season generously with salt and pepper and mix well. Cover the container and put it in the refrigerator to marinate for at least 3 hours.

4. Serve as a dip with crunchy vegetables. Any leftover shrimp salsa can be stored in the refrigerator for up to 3 days.

Nutritional analysis per serving (1 cup): calories 195, fat 10 g, saturated fat 1.5 g, cholesterol 0 mg, fiber 7.1 g, protein 14 g, carbohydrate 16.3 g, sodium 289 mg

Mexican Shrimp "Ceviche"

Serves: 6

Prep time:
20 minutes

Cook time:
5 minutes

Chill time:
3 hours

Level: Easy

Budget: $$

Ceviche is a spicy, delicious way to eat fish. Shrimp is a wonderful source of protein, very low in toxins, and is delightful when prepared this way. This dish contains cooked shrimp and so is not technically a ceviche, but it tastes just like one.

- 1 pound raw shrimp, peeled and deveined
- ½ medium white onion, finely chopped
- 1 large tomato, finely chopped
- ¼ cup tomato sauce
- juice of 4 limes
- 2 teaspoons hot pepper sauce
- ½ bunch (about 1 ½ ounces) fresh cilantro, finely chopped
- 2 avocados, peeled, pitted, and roughly chopped
- ½ large head green cabbage, finely shredded
- 2 limes, cut into wedges

1. In a saucepan, bring about 2 quarts of water to a boil over high heat. Add the shrimp (add water if necessary so shrimp are covered with 1 inch of water) and cook until just pink, 2–3 minutes.

2. Drain the cooked shrimp and transfer them to a large bowl of ice water to stop them from cooking further. When cool, drain and chop them into bite-size pieces.

3. Transfer the shrimp to a large nonreactive container and add the onion, tomato, tomato sauce, lime juice, hot pepper sauce, and cilantro and mix well until evenly combined. Taste for seasoning and adjust if needed with additional salt, lime juice, or hot pepper sauce.

4. Cover the container and let the ceviche marinate in the refrigerator for 2–3 hours. Serve each portion on a small bed of shredded cabbage,

with lime wedges alongside. Any leftover ceviche can be stored in the refrigerator for up to 2 days.

Nutritional analysis per serving (1 cup): calories 215, fat 11 g, saturated fat 2 g, cholesterol 147 mg, fiber 7 g, protein 20 g, carbohydrate 13 g, sodium 302 mg

ADDICTIVE CREAMY GARLIC DRESSING

Serves: 12

Prep time:
10 minutes

Level: Easy

Budget: $

This delicious protein-rich dressing can be used on salad or as a dip for meat, chicken, or vegetables. Garlic is a fabulous immune-boosting, antimicrobial, blood-pressure-lowering, cholesterol-optimizing food.

- 1 cup macadamia nuts
- sea salt and freshly ground black pepper to taste
- ¼ teaspoon dry mustard
- 4 garlic cloves, minced
- 2 tablespoons apple cider vinegar
- 2 tablespoons red wine vinegar
- ⅓ cup water
- ⅔ cup extra-virgin olive oil

Combine all of the ingredients except the oil in a blender and blend on high speed for 1 minute. Slowly drizzle in the oil and blend until the dressing is smooth and creamy. Check for seasoning and add more salt or black pepper if desired. The dressing can be refrigerated for up to 5 days.

Nutritional analysis per serving (2 tablespoons): calories 188, fat 21 g, saturated fat 3 g, cholesterol 0 mg, fiber 1 g, protein 1 g, carbohydrate 2 g, sodium 40 mg

ARTICHOKE HEARTS WITH CARAMELIZED ONIONS AND HERB DRESSING

This delicious side dish is best prepared ahead and makes a great addition to an antipasto platter.

- 1 (9-ounce) can artichoke hearts, rinsed and drained
- ¼ cup extra-virgin olive oil
- 4 garlic cloves, minced
- ¼ teaspoon red pepper flakes
- ¼ teaspoon paprika
- 2 teaspoons finely chopped fresh parsley
- 2 teaspoons finely chopped fresh tarragon
- 2 large red onions, finely sliced
- 2 large yellow onions, finely sliced
- juice of ½ large lemon

Serves: 4

Prep time: 15 minutes

Cook time: 50 minutes

Level: Easy

Budget: $

1. Preheat the oven to 350°F.
2. In a small bowl, combine the artichokes with 2 tablespoons of the olive oil, the garlic, spices, and herbs, and toss until evenly mixed.
3. Spread out the mixture onto a baking sheet and roast until the artichokes are soft and brown, 30–35 minutes, turning throughout to evenly cook. Be careful not to burn them.
4. Heat the remaining 2 tablespoons olive oil in a medium cast-iron pan over medium heat. After a minute add the onions and cook until soft, 5–6 minutes. Reduce the heat to low and continue to cook, stirring occasionally to prevent them from burning, until well caramelized, 15–20 minutes.
5. Stir in the lemon juice and cook for another minute.
6. In a large bowl, combine the roasted artichokes and caramelized onion mixture. Gently mix until everything is evenly combined.

7. Serve warm or at room temperature. Any leftover artichokes can be refrigerated for up to 4 days.

Nutritional analysis per serving (½ cup): calories 211, fat 14 g, saturated fat 2 g, cholesterol 0 mg, fiber 4 g, protein 3 g, carbohydrate 21 g, sodium 218 mg

ASPARAGUS WITH ROASTED GARLIC, OLIVE OIL, AND RED ONIONS

Serves: 4

Prep time: 15 minutes

Cook time: 35 minutes

Level: Easy

Budget: $

The fresh herbs balance out the deep, pungent flavor of the roasted garlic. This is the perfect side dish to complement any chicken or fish entrée.

- 1 head garlic, halved
- 1½ tablespoons extra-virgin olive oil
- 1 medium red onion, finely sliced
- ½ teaspoon sea salt
- ¼ teaspoon cayenne pepper
- 1 teaspoon minced fresh thyme
- 1 teaspoon minced fresh basil
- 1 teaspoon minced fresh parsley
- 1 pound asparagus, trimmed

1. Preheat the oven to 325°F.

2. Split the garlic head in half and brush it all over with ½ tablespoon of the oil. Put the halves back together and wrap the garlic loosely in foil. Place the head of garlic on a baking sheet and roast in the oven for 30 minutes. Let cool.

3. Heat ½ tablespoon of the oil in a medium sauté pan over medium heat. Add the onion and cook until it caramelizes, 10–12 minutes.

4. When the garlic is cool enough to handle, squeeze out all the soft roasted garlic into a medium bowl. Add the salt, cayenne pepper, herbs, and remaining ½ tablespoon oil, and combine with a spoon, mashing the garlic as you mix.

5. Bring a pot of water to a boil over high heat. When it boils, cook the asparagus in the water until tender, 3–4 minutes.

6. Drain the asparagus and transfer to the bowl with the garlic and herb mixture, and toss until well coated. Pour out the contents of the bowl

onto a platter and top with the caramelized onions. The asparagus is best when served hot but can be refrigerated for up to 3 days.

Nutritional analysis per serving (½ cup): calories 147, fat 7 g, saturated fat 1 g, cholesterol 0 mg, fiber 3 g, protein 4 g, carbohydrate 20 g, sodium 109 mg

ASPARAGUS WITH ROASTED SHALLOTS AND CAYENNE PEPPER

Serves: 4

Prep time: 15 minutes

Cook time: 40 minutes

Level: Easy

Budget: $

Roasting the shallots brings out their inherent sweetness. The addition of the cayenne perks this up with just enough spice. This delicious side dish is low-glycemic and will please the entire family.

- 4 shallots, peeled
- 2 tablespoons extra-virgin olive oil
- 1 pound asparagus, trimmed
- 2 teaspoons finely chopped fresh basil
- 1 teaspoon finely chopped fresh thyme
- ½ teaspoon cayenne pepper
- ½ teaspoon sea salt

1. Preheat the oven to 350 °F.
2. Put the shallots in a small roasting pan and drizzle 1 tablespoon of the oil over them.
3. Put the pan in the oven on the bottom rack and roast until the shallots are golden brown and soft, 25–30 minutes. Toss them occasionally during the cooking so that they brown evenly. When cooked, remove the shallots, slice them thickly, and transfer to a small bowl.
4. Bring a pot of water to boil over high heat. Cook the asparagus until tender, 3–4 minutes. Drain well and arrange on a platter.
5. Add the remaining 1 tablespoon olive oil, herbs, cayenne pepper, and salt to the shallots and gently toss to combine. Pour the roasted shallot mixture over the asparagus and serve. The asparagus is best when served hot but can be refrigerated for up to 3 days.

Nutritional analysis per serving (½ cup): calories 110, fat 6 g, saturated fat 1 g, cholesterol 0 mg, fiber 2 g, protein 3 g, carbohydrate 13 g, sodium 109 mg

BROCCOLI WITH SAUTÉED CARROTS

Serves: 4

Prep time:
15 minutes

Cook time:
15 minutes

Level: Easy

Budget: $

Blanching the broccoli ensures a bright green color, which is a gorgeous accent to this dish. Use turmeric to add both color and protective antioxidants.

- 1 medium head broccoli, cut into small florets
- 2 teaspoons extra-virgin olive oil
- 2 large carrots, peeled and cut on the bias into ¼-inch slices
- ½ teaspoon sea salt
- 1 teaspoon finely chopped fresh parsley
- ½ teaspoon finely chopped fresh thyme
- ¼ teaspoon onion powder
- ¼ teaspoon ground turmeric
- ⅛ teaspoon cayenne pepper

1. Bring a small pot of water to a boil over high heat. Blanch the broccoli until it turns a brighter shade of green, 2–3 minutes.

2. Heat the oil in a large sauté pan over medium heat. When hot, add the carrots, season them with the salt, and cook for 5–6 minutes.

3. Add the blanched broccoli and all the herbs and spices. Toss the carrots and broccoli in the spices and cook until the carrots are tender, 5-7 minutes. Serve hot or at room temperature. Any leftover broccoli and carrots can be refrigerated for up to 4 days.

Nutritional analysis per serving (½ cup): calories 86, fat 3 g, saturated fat 0 g, cholesterol 0 mg, fiber 5 g, protein 5 g, carbohydrate 13 g, sodium 309 mg

BROCCOLINI WITH HOT PEPPERS AND GARLIC

Broccolini is part of the Brassica family. It is similar to broccoli in taste and nutrition but has slightly smaller florets and longer, spinier stems. The poblano pepper makes this dish burst with flavor and a hint of spice.

- 1 tablespoon extra-virgin olive oil
- 1 medium poblano pepper, seeded and thinly sliced
- 4 garlic cloves, thinly sliced
- ½ large shallot, minced
- 2 medium bunches broccolini, cut into 2-inch pieces
- ½ teaspoon sea salt

Serves: 4

Prep time: 10 minutes

Cook time: 10 minutes

Level: Easy

Budget: $

1. Heat the oil in a large sauté pan over medium heat. After a minute, add the pepper, garlic, and shallot, and sauté them for 1–2 minutes.

2. Add the broccolini and sauté until tender but still slightly crisp, 3–4 minutes. Season with the salt and mix until the salt is evenly distributed.

3. Remove the pan from the heat and transfer the broccolini to a platter. Serve hot. Leftover greens can be refrigerated for up to 4 days.

Nutritional analysis per serving (½ cup): calories 58, fat 3 g, saturated fat 0 g, cholesterol 0 mg, fiber 4 g, protein 4 g, carbohydrate 69 g, sodium 140 mg

Learn to Love Brussels Sprouts

Serves: 3

Prep time: 5 minutes

Cook time: 20 minutes

Level: Easy

Budget: $

Despite many people's fear of Brussels sprouts, when prepared carefully and cooked properly, they can be delicious. They are also an extraordinary super-food rich in glucosinolates, antioxidants, folate, and other metabolism-boosting nutrients.

- 2 tablespoons extra-virgin olive oil
- 2 garlic cloves, minced
- 1 small leek (white part only), thinly sliced
- sea salt and freshly ground black pepper
- 1 pound Brussels sprouts, trimmed and halved
- ¼ cup balsamic vinegar

1. Heat the oil in a wok or large cast-iron pan over medium heat. When the oil is almost smoking, add the garlic and stir-fry it until aromatic, about 1 minute. Toss in the leek and season to taste with salt and black pepper. Stir-fry until the leek has softened, about 3 minutes.

2. Add the Brussels sprouts and pour in the balsamic vinegar. Stir-fry until the vinegar has glazed the Brussels sprouts nicely, about 5 minutes. Serve hot. Any leftover Brussels sprouts can be stored the refrigerator for up to 4 days.

Nutritional analysis per serving (1 cup): calories 170, fat 10 g, saturated fat 1 g, cholesterol 0 mg, fiber 6 g, protein 6 g, carbohydrate 19 g, sodium 45 mg

CARROT, HOT PEPPER, AND SHALLOT STIR-FRY WITH GINGER AND GARLIC

Serves: 4

Prep time: 15 minutes

Cook time: 15 minutes

Level: Easy

Budget: $

This is one of the most exciting dishes and a treat for your senses. The Chinese 5-spice powder gives you all five taste sensations—sweet, salty, bitter, sour and umami. This dish is sure to please.

- 1 tablespoon extra-virgin olive oil
- 4 cups baby carrots
- 3 shallots, thinly sliced
- 2 garlic cloves, minced
- ½-inch piece fresh ginger, peeled and minced
- ½ small jalapeño pepper, seeded and minced
- ½ teaspoon Chinese 5-spice powder
- 1 teaspoon sea salt
- ¼ teaspoon red pepper flakes
- 3 scallions, finely sliced

1. Heat the olive oil in a large sauté pan over medium-high heat. When hot, add the carrots and shallots. Sauté for 4–5 minutes, then add the garlic, ginger, jalapeño, 5-spice powder, salt, and red pepper flakes and stir until well mixed.

2. Sauté for 4–5 more minutes, turn off the heat, and add the scallions. The carrots should be tender but still crisp in the center. Serve hot or at room temperature. Any leftover carrots can be refrigerated for up to 5 days.

Nutritional analysis per serving (1 cup): calories 86, fat 4 g, saturated fat 0 g, cholesterol 0 mg, fiber 2 g, protein 1 g, carbohydrate 13 g, sodium 346 mg

ASIAN COLESLAW

Serves: 4

Prep time:
5 minutes

Chill time:
30 minutes

Level: Easy

Budget: $

This salad is easy to make and tastes wonderful with a little added shrimp or grilled chicken.

- 1 large head green cabbage, finely shredded
- ½ small head red cabbage, finely shredded
- 1 large carrot, peeled and finely shredded
- 2 teaspoons toasted sesame oil
- 3 tablespoons extra-virgin olive oil
- 6 scallions, finely sliced
- ½ bunch (about 1½ ounces) fresh cilantro, roughly chopped
- juice of 2 limes
- sea salt
- ½ cup chopped roasted unsalted cashews

1. Mix the green and red cabbages with the carrots in a large bowl.
2. In a small bowl whisk together the sesame oil, olive oil, scallions, cilantro, and lime juice, and season to taste with salt. Pour the mixture over the cabbage and toss well.
3. Let the slaw sit in the refrigerator for at least 30 minutes. Garnish with cashews before serving. Any leftovers can be stored in the refrigerator for up to 4 days.

Nutritional analysis per serving (½ cup): calories 43, fat 10 g, saturated fat 2 g, cholesterol 0 mg, fiber 2 g, protein 2 g, carbohydrate 6 g, sodium 39 mg

ROASTED CAULIFLOWER

Roasting vegetables brings out their sweet, crunchy flavor. This is a perfect hors d'oeuvre or kid-friendly vegetable surprise.

- 2 tablespoons extra-virgin olive oil
- 1 tablespoon ground cumin
- 2 teaspoons curry powder
- ½ teaspoon cayenne pepper
- ¼ teaspoon sea salt
- 1 large head cauliflower, cut into large florets

Serves: 4

Prep time: 5 minutes

Cook time: 30 minutes

Level: Easy

Budget: $

1. Preheat the oven to 375°F.
2. In a large bowl whisk together the olive oil, cumin, curry powder, cayenne pepper, and salt. Add the cauliflower to the bowl and toss until it's evenly coated in the spice oil.
3. Dump the cauliflower onto a baking sheet or roasting pan and drizzle on any spice oil that was left behind in the bowl.
4. Roast for 25–30 minutes, stirring once after 15 minutes. When done the cauliflower should be tender and browned in spots. Let cool for 5 minutes before serving. Any leftover cauliflower can be stored in the refrigerator for up to 4 days.

Note: You can substitute any combination of fresh herbs, dried herbs, or spices for the ones in this recipe. If using fresh herbs, increase to 3 tablespoons.

Nutritional analysis per serving (1 cup): calories 174, fat 15 g, saturated fat 2 g, cholesterol 14 mg, fiber 5 g, protein 4 g, carbohydrate 10 g, sodium 47 mg

CAULIFLOWER MASHED PSEUDO-POTATOES

Serves: 3
Prep time: 10 minutes
Cook time: 25 minutes
Level: Easy
Budget: $

You will never miss mashed potatoes once you try this yummy cauliflower substitute. And you get all of the healthful benefits of the vegetables, spices, and flavors in this dish.

- 1 tablespoon extra-virgin olive oil
- 1 medium head cauliflower, cut into large florets, stem sliced ½-inch thick
- 1 medium apple, peeled and cored, chopped
- 1 medium yellow onion, chopped
- 2 teaspoons curry powder
- sea salt and freshly ground black pepper
- 1 cup water

1. Heat the oil in a large cast-iron pan over medium heat. When the oil is shimmering, add the cauliflower, apple, onion, and curry powder. Season to taste with salt and black pepper and mix well until the cauliflower is coated in the oil and spices. Cook, stirring frequently, for 8 minutes.

2. Turn the heat down to low and add the water. Cover and cook until the cauliflower is completely tender, 10–15 minutes.

3. Transfer the contents of the pan to a food processor and pulse the cauliflower mixture until it is creamy but thick, similar to the consistency of mashed potatoes. Add a little more water if necessary, but be careful or you'll wind up with cauliflower soup.

4. Check for seasoning and add more salt and pepper if necessary. Any leftover mashed cauliflower can be stored in the refrigerator for up to 4 days.

Nutritional analysis per serving (1 cup): calories 215, fat 11 g, saturated fat 2 g, cholesterol 147 mg, fiber 7 g, protein 20 g, carbohydrate 13 g, sodium 226 mg

MOROCCAN SPICED GREEN BEANS WITH SHALLOTS

This is a quick and easy side dish to accompany your main meal. Lightly sautéing the green beans helps them retain their natural crisp texture. The cilantro and mint add freshness to this savory dish.

- 1 tablespoon extra-virgin olive oil
- 1 pound green beans, trimmed
- 1 shallot, diced
- ¼ teaspoon ground cumin
- 2 teaspoons chopped fresh cilantro
- 1 teaspoon chopped fresh mint
- 1 teaspoon chopped fresh parsley
- ¼ teaspoon paprika
- ¼ teaspoon red pepper flakes
- 1 teaspoon sea salt

Serves: 4

Prep time: 10 minutes

Cook time: 10 minutes

Level: Easy

Budget: $

1. Heat the oil in a large sauté pan over medium-high heat. Add the green beans and shallot and sauté until they begin to soften, 2–3 minutes.

2. Add all of the seasonings and toss the beans to coat them evenly. Continue to cook until the beans are tender but firm, 2–3 minutes. Serve warm or chilled. Leftover beans can be refrigerated for up to 5 days.

Nutritional analysis per serving (½ cup): calories 70, fat 4 g, saturated fat 1 g, cholesterol 0 mg, fiber 4 g, protein 2 g, carbohydrate 9 g, sodium 476 mg

KALE AND BRUSSELS SPROUT SALAD

Serves: 4

Prep time: 10 minutes

Cook time: 5 minutes

Level: Easy

Budget: $

Every day I try to include something from the broccoli family, and this kale and Brussels sprout salad is a fabulous surprise for many people. This should help you to break out of your routine.

ALMOND GARNISH:

- ¼ cup slivered almonds

DRESSING:

- juice of 2 lemons
- 1 tablespoon Dijon mustard
- ½ small shallot
- 1 garlic clove
- ½ teaspoon sea salt
- ¼ teaspoon freshly ground black pepper
- ¼ cup extra-virgin olive oil

KALE AND BRUSSELS SPROUTS:

- 1 large bunch kale, stemmed and thinly sliced
- ½ pound Brussels sprouts, trimmed and thinly sliced

TOAST THE ALMONDS:

1. Preheat the oven to 350°F.
2. Toast the almond slivers on an ungreased baking sheet until light brown, 5–8 minutes. Cool and reserve.

MAKE THE DRESSING:

Combine all of the dressing ingredients except the oil in a blender. Blend on high speed for 1 minute while slowly pouring in the oil. Taste for seasoning and add more salt and black pepper if needed.

ASSEMBLE THE SALAD:

Spoon a few tablespoons of the dressing around the sides of a large salad bowl. Add the kale and Brussels sprouts and toss gently to coat everything evenly. Garnish with the almonds. Leftover dressing can be stored in the refrigerator for up to 5 days. Stir or shake before using.

Nutritional analysis per serving (1 cup): calories 265, fat 20 g, saturated fat 3 g, cholesterol 0 mg, fiber 5 g, protein 8 g, carbohydrate 20 g, sodium 163 mg

SEASONED KALE

Serves: 4

Prep time:
5 minutes

Cook time:
35 minutes

Level: Easy

Budget: $

Kale is an inexpensive superfood available throughout the year. I grow it from April through December in my garden and I live in the northeast! Kale is full of folate, magnesium, and other wonderful disease- and fat-busting ingredients. Learning how to prepare kale well will allow you to get your daily dose of powerful detoxifiers.

- 3 tablespoons extra-virgin olive oil
- 1 small red onion, thinly sliced
- 2 garlic cloves, minced
- 1 tablespoon hot pepper sauce
- 1 tablespoon red wine vinegar
- 1½ large bunches kale, stemmed and roughly chopped
- sea salt and freshly ground black pepper

1. Heat the oil in a large pot over medium heat. When the oil is hot, add the onion. Cook, stirring frequently, until it softens and begins to caramelize, about 4 minutes.

2. Add the garlic to the pot and cook until aromatic, about 1 minute. Add the hot pepper sauce and vinegar.

3. Toss the kale into the pot and season to taste with salt and pepper. Reduce the heat to medium-low and cook until the kale is completely tender and wilted, 20–30 minutes. Check for seasoning and adjust with more salt, pepper, or vinegar if needed. Any leftover kale can be stored in the refrigerator for up to 4 days.

Nutritional analysis per serving (½ cup): calories 155, fat 11 g, saturated fat 2 g, cholesterol 280 mg, fiber 4 g, protein 4 g, carbohydrate 13 g, sodium 236 mg

KALE WITH CARROTS AND ARAME

Seaweed is an important vegetable to add to your diet because it is rich in minerals and is a powerful heavy-metal detoxifier. It is also a good source of iodine, which your thyroid needs, and it helps you easily absorb calcium and magnesium. This staple of Asian diets is foreign to many of us but worth the adventure.

- ¼ cup dried arame seaweed
- 3 cups water
- 2 tablespoons extra-virgin olive oil
- 3 medium carrots, peeled and sliced
- 3 garlic cloves, minced
- sea salt
- red pepper flakes
- 1 large bunch kale, stemmed and roughly chopped

Serves: 6

Prep time: 35 minutes

Cook time: 15 minutes

Level: Easy

Budget: $

1. Place the arame in a large bowl and cover with the water. Let soak for 30 minutes. Drain the arame and rinse it thoroughly with fresh cold water. Squeeze out the excess moisture and place in a clean bowl.

2. Heat the oil in a wok or large cast-iron pan over medium heat. When the oil is almost smoking, add the carrots and cook, stirring frequently, for 3 minutes. Add the garlic and cook for 1 minute.

3. Toss in the seaweed, season to taste with salt and red pepper flakes, and stir until mixed well.

4. Add the kale and stir-fry it with the carrots, seaweed, and garlic for 5–6 minutes. It should still be slightly crunchy but mostly cooked through. Check for seasoning and add more salt and red pepper flakes if needed. Any leftover kale can be stored in the refrigerator for up to 4 days.

Nutritional analysis per serving (⅓ cup): calories 94, fat 7 g, saturated fat 1 g, cholesterol 0 mg, fiber 2 g, protein 2 g, carbohydrate 8 g, sodium 123 mg

GRILLED MIXED VEGETABLES

Serves: 8

Prep time:
15 minutes

Cook time:
30 minutes

Level: Easy

Budget: $

Grilling vegetables enhances their wonderful flavor. You can make large quantities of grilled vegetables, store them in the fridge, and have them available for quick, easy snacks.

- 1 large eggplant, thickly sliced
- 3 medium zucchini, thickly sliced
- 2 large red bell peppers, seeded and thickly sliced
- 1 large green bell pepper, seeded and thickly sliced
- 2 large onions, thickly sliced
- 1 pound asparagus
- 2 large tomatoes, thickly sliced
- 3 tablespoons extra-virgin olive oil
- sea salt and freshly ground black pepper to taste

1. Preheat the grill. Liberally brush the vegetables with 2½ tablespoons of the olive oil and season them to taste with salt and black pepper.

2. Once the grates are hot lay on all of the vegetables. Flip often and watch them closely to make sure they don't burn.

3. Grill the vegetables until they are soft and lightly charred, 8–10 minutes. Transfer to a platter and drizzle with the remaining ½ tablespoon olive oil. Any leftover vegetables can be stored in the refrigerator for up to 4 days. Eat cold or reheat in a low oven before serving.

Nutritional analysis per serving (1 cup): calories 84, fat 4 g, saturated fat 1 g, cholesterol 0 mg, fiber 5 g, protein 3 g, carbohydrate 12 g, sodium 11 mg

SPECIAL BEANS AND GREENS

Mediterranean cooking is a great way to eat for reversing diabesity. The low-fat, high-fiber beans in this dish keep your blood sugar stable all day. The garlic not only is tasty and smells great while cooking, but it is a wonderful way to reduce inflammation.

Serves: 6

Prep time: 15 minutes

Cook time: 1 hour

Level: Moderate

Budget: $

- 4 red bell peppers
- 2 tablespoons extra-virgin olive oil
- 3 garlic cloves, minced
- sea salt and freshly ground black pepper
- 1 pound baby spinach
- 4 cups cooked cannellini beans or 2 (15-ounce) cans cannellini beans, rinsed and drained
- 1 cup low-sodium chicken or vegetable broth
- juice of 1 small lemon

1. Rub the peppers with 1 tablespoon of the oil and roast them over an open flame, on a grill, or in the oven under the broiler element until the skin is completely charred. Place the peppers in a bowl and cover tightly with plastic wrap. Let sit for 5 minutes, peel away all blackened skin, and remove the seeds and stems. (To save time, use jarred roasted red peppers.)

2. Heat the remaining 1 tablespoon oil in a large cast-iron pan over medium heat. After a minute or two add the garlic to the pan. Cook, stirring, until the garlic is aromatic, 2–3 minutes.

3. Stir in the roasted red peppers and season to taste with salt and black pepper. Add the spinach, beans, and broth and cover the pan. Cook until the spinach has wilted and the beans are hot, about 5 minutes. Turn off the heat and stir in the lemon juice. Check for seasoning and add more salt or black pepper if desired.

4. Transfer the beans and greens to a platter and serve immediately. Any leftovers can be stored in the refrigerator for up to 5 days.

Nutritional analysis per serving (1 cup): calories 142, fat 3 g, saturated fat 0 g, cholesterol 0 mg, fiber 7 g, protein 8 g, carbohydrate 23 g, sodium 152 mg

6

Reintroduction

Food is your friend, not your foe. But certain foods can trigger undesirable reactions that make you fatigued, fat, foggy, or worse. These are food sensitivities. Other foods, like sugar, can trigger neurobiological addiction and reawaken old habits of cravings and bingeing. Your body is the best barometer of what works for you and what doesn't. The Basic and Advanced Plans eliminate the two most common food sensitivities from your diet—dairy and gluten—and all forms of sugar.

But after 6–12 weeks of following the principles of the Blood Sugar Solution, many of you will have rebooted and reset your metabolism and your immune system. That is why I encourage you to experiment carefully with reintroducing gluten and dairy into your diet. Follow the guidelines on page 58 to help you get started with the reintroduction process. Use the food log on page 61, and be sure to read Chapter 26 in *The Blood Sugar Solution* for a comprehensive explanation of the process of reintroducing common food allergens. Try the recipes in this chapter during your reintroduction phase. Remember, if you are sensitive to gluten or dairy, continuing to eat it will only delay your healing and recovery. When in doubt, leave it out!

BREAKFAST

RAW CHOCOLATE PROTEIN SHAKE

Serves: 2

Prep time:
5 minutes

Level: Easy

Budget: $

This simple creamy shake is easy to make and will start your day off with adequate protein. It is also a good source of chocolate, which contains special fats that help improve your metabolism. And it tastes great! Protein powder is a nutrition supplement to add additional protein to a meal or shake. Look for a plant-based protein powder made from chia, hemp, or rice protein.

- 1 frozen banana, roughly chopped
- 1½ ounces chocolate protein powder
- 2 tablespoons unsweetened cacao powder
- 1 cup unsweetened almond milk
- ½ teaspoon pure vanilla extract
- ½ cup ice cubes
- 1 cup baby spinach

Combine all of the ingredients in a blender. Blend on high speed until the ice is crushed and the drink is smooth, about 2 minutes. If the shake is too thick, add a little more almond milk and blend again. Serve immediately.

Nutritional analysis per serving (1 cup): calories 246, fat 3 g, saturated fat 1 g, cholesterol 0 mg, fiber 8 g, protein 19 g, carbohydrate 36 g, sodium 255 mg

MAKE-AHEAD SUPER WARM AND FILLING BREAKFAST

Oatmeal can raise your blood sugar; however, nuts and coconut help to balance the glycemic load of this breakfast. The sweet Vidalia onions provide a sweet-savory touch to this traditional breakfast food.

Serves: 6
Prep time: 10 minutes
Cook time: 15 minutes
Level: Easy
Budget: $$

- 1 cup steel-cut oats
- ¼ small Vidalia onion, finely chopped
- 4 cups water
- sea salt
- ½ cup chopped raw almonds
- ½ cup chopped raw pecans
- ½ cup chopped raw walnuts
- ½ cup ground flaxseeds
- 1 cup unsweetened coconut milk
- 1 cup unsweetened shredded coconut

1. Add the oats, onion, and water to a medium pot and place over high heat. When it reaches a boil, reduce the heat to low. Season with a pinch of salt and simmer with the lid slightly ajar for 8–10 minutes.

2. Remove the lid and add the nuts and ground flaxseeds. Cover the pot and cook for 5 minutes longer.

3. Take the pot off the heat and stir in the coconut milk. Garnish with shredded coconut. Serve right away or transfer to a bowl and store in the refrigerator for up to 3 days.

Nutritional analysis per serving (1 cup): calories 324, fat 27 g, saturated fat 10 g, cholesterol 0 mg, fiber 7 g, protein 8 g, carbohydrate 10 g, sodium 300 mg

EGGWICH

Serves: 1

Prep time:
10 minutes

Cook time:
15 minutes

Level: Easy

Budget: $

This protein-packed breakfast is a quick and creative take on a traditional omelet. The green from the avocado complements the other vegetable colors peeking out from the eggs. Look for gluten-free bread made from whole-grain and nut-based flours.

- 1 teaspoon extra-virgin olive oil
- 2 large egg whites
- sea salt and freshly ground black pepper
- 1 roasted red bell pepper (jarred or freshly roasted), seeded and chopped
- 1 shiitake mushroom, stemmed and thickly sliced
- ½ large kale leaf, stemmed and roughly chopped
- 2 tablespoons feta cheese, crumbled
- ½ teaspoon ground turmeric
- 1 slice gluten-free bread
- ½ avocado, peeled, pitted, and mashed

1. Preheat the oven to 400°F.
2. Pour the oil and egg whites into an 8-ounce ramekin. Season the eggs to taste with salt and black pepper and add the roasted pepper, mushrooms, kale, cheese, and turmeric. Place the ramekin on a small baking sheet and slide the sheet into the oven on the top rack. Bake until the eggs have puffed and are set, 12–15 minutes.
3. While the eggs cook, toast the bread, slice it in half, and evenly spread the mashed avocado over both sides.
4. Remove the ramekin from the oven and turn the eggs and vegetables out onto one of the bread halves. Top with the other bread half and serve while hot.

Nutritional analysis per serving (1 eggwich): calories 266, fat 13 g, saturated fat 0 g, cholesterol 0 mg, fiber 6 g, protein 6 g, carbohydrate 37 g, sodium 401 mg

BROCCOLI SCRAMBLE

The broccoli provides a phytonutrient called DIM, which is helpful in estrogen metabolism. Using one whole egg and the whites from three more eggs is a great way to maximize protein and healthy omega-3 fats without losing the potent antioxidant lutein from the yolk.

- 2 teaspoons extra-virgin olive oil
- ½ medium Vidalia onion, roughly chopped
- 2 cups broccoli, cut into small florets
- sea salt and freshly ground black pepper
- 1 large egg
- 3 large egg whites
- 1 tablespoon finely grated Parmigiano Reggiano cheese
- 2 slices gluten-free bread, toasted

Serves: 2

Prep time: 5 minutes

Cook time: 15

Level: Easy

Budget: $

1. Heat the oil in a medium nonstick pan over medium heat. Add the onion and cook until translucent, about 4 minutes.

2. Add the broccoli. Season to taste with salt and black pepper and cook, stirring occasionally, until bright green and soft, 5–6 minutes.

3. Combine the egg and egg whites in a small bowl and beat until well mixed. Add the eggs to the pan with the broccoli and cook until completely scrambled, 2-3 minutes.

4. Turn off the heat and sprinkle on the cheese. Toss the scramble until evenly mixed and divide between two plates. Serve each with a slice of toasted gluten-free bread.

Nutritional analysis per serving (½ the scramble and 1 slice gluten-free bread): calories 271, fat 12 g, saturated fat 4 g, cholesterol 84 mg, fiber 4 g, protein 14 g, carbohydrate 29 g, sodium 613 mg

SPICY SAGE TURKEY SAUSAGE

Serves: 4

Prep time: 5 minutes

Cook time: 15 minutes

Level: Easy

Budget: $$

Sage accents the sausage beautifully to create the comforting savory taste of a hearty breakfast. Serve with eggs over greens to make a complete meal.

- 2 cups cooked jasmine rice
- 1 pound lean ground turkey
- 1 large egg plus 1 large egg white
- ⅓ cup rolled oats
- 4 scallions, finely sliced
- 1 teaspoon dried sage
- ¼ teaspoon dried rosemary
- ¼ teaspoon dried thyme
- ¼ teaspoon red pepper flakes
- sea salt and freshly ground black pepper to taste
- 2 tablespoons extra-virgin olive oil

1. Combine all of the ingredients except the oil in a large bowl and mix until the spices are evenly incorporated.
2. Heat the oil in a large cast-iron pan over medium-high heat. Once hot, add a marble-sized piece of the sausage to see if it's properly seasoned. Cook for a couple of minutes on each side until brown and then taste. Add more salt or black pepper to the sausage base if desired.
3. Divide the sausage into 4 patties and lay the patties in the hot oil.
4. Cook until brown, about 4 minutes per side. You can store any uncooked sausage meat tightly in the refrigerator for up to 4 days or in the freezer for up to 2 months.

Nutritional analysis per serving (1 patty): calories 170, fat 3 g, saturated fat 1 g, cholesterol 95 mg, fiber 1 g, protein 30 g, carbohydrate 6 g, sodium 682 mg

SOUPS

CURRIED WINTER SQUASH SOUP

Serves: 8

Prep time: 15 minutes

Cook time: 40 minutes

Level: Easy

Budget: $

The secret ingredient in this delicious winter squash soup is tahini paste, which is rich in calcium and healthy fats, and has a creamy curry flavor that adds a unique spiciness to the soup. Curry and squash are one of my favorite combinations.

- 1 large butternut squash, peeled, seeded, and chopped
- 1 large delicata squash, peeled, seeded, and chopped
- 2 tablespoons extra-virgin olive oil
- sea salt and freshly ground black pepper
- 3 tablespoons grapeseed oil
- 1 large shallot, finely chopped
- 3 garlic cloves, minced
- 1 tablespoon plus 1 teaspoon curry powder
- ½ teaspoon ground cumin
- 1 tablespoon tahini paste
- 3 cups unsweetened almond milk

1. Preheat the oven to 400°F.

2. Toss the squash in a large bowl with the olive oil. Season it generously with salt and black pepper and pour out onto one or two large baking sheets or roasting pans in a single layer. Roast until light brown and tender, about 30 minutes.

3. While the squash roasts, heat the grapeseed oil in a medium pot over medium heat. Sauté the shallot and garlic for 3 minutes, then stir in the curry powder and cumin. Cook for 2 more minutes, then transfer the mixture to a blender.

4. Remove the squash from the oven and add it to the blender along with the tahini and almond milk. Blend on high speed until smooth. Check for seasoning and add salt or black pepper if desired. Serve hot.

Any leftovers can be stored in the refrigerator for up to 5 days or in the freezer for up to 6 months.

Nutritional analysis per serving (1 cup): calories 183, fat 10 g, saturated fat 1 g, cholesterol 0 mg, fiber 4 g, protein 3 g, carbohydrate 22 g, sodium 139 mg

SALADS

KICKIN' KALE SALAD

This is a delicious and easy way to eat more kale. The artichokes provide flavor as well as silymarin, which helps increase your liver's ability to detoxify.

Serves: 6

Prep time: 5 minutes

Level: Easy

Budget: $

DRESSING:

- juice of ½ large lemon
- 3 tablespoons extra-virgin olive oil
- sea salt and freshly ground black pepper

SALAD:

- 1 medium bunch kale, chopped
- 2 large roasted red bell peppers (jarred or freshly roasted), seeded and chopped
- ½ medium red onion, finely chopped
- 2 garlic cloves, minced
- 1 cup cooked cannellini beans or ½ (15-ounce) can cannellini beans, rinsed and drained
- 12 ounces fresh, canned, or thawed frozen artichoke hearts
- 1 cup black olives, pitted and halved
- 8 ounces fresh mozzarella, diced

MAKE THE DRESSING:

In a small bowl whisk the vinegar while slowly adding the olive oil. Season to taste with salt and pepper. Whisk until the dressing has thickened slightly.

ASSEMBLE THE SALAD:

Combine all of the salad ingredients in a medium bowl and toss until the greens and beans are evenly distributed. Spoon over the dressing and give the salad another toss until everything is well coated in dressing. Serve immediately.

Nutritional analysis per serving (1 cup): calories 317, fat 6 g, saturated fat 1 g, cholesterol 0 mg, fiber 11 g, protein 18 g, carbohydrate 54 g, sodium 379 mg

EDAMAME BEAN SALAD

This salad is a great way to enjoy whole-soy foods. Edamame are rich in fiber, complete protein, and phytoestrogens. The bright red tomatoes are a colorful addition to the salad and complement the earthy tones of the beans.

Serves: 12

Prep time: 5 minutes

Level: Easy

Budget: $

DRESSING:

- juice of 1 large lime
- 1 garlic clove, minced
- sea salt and freshly ground black pepper to taste
- 2 tablespoons extra-virgin olive oil

SALAD:

- 1 medium bunch kale, stemmed and chopped
- 2 large roasted red peppers (jarred or freshly roasted), seeded and chopped
- ½ medium red onion, finely chopped
- 2 garlic cloves, minced
- 2 cup cooked black beans or 1 (15-ounce) can black beans, rinsed and drained
- 2 cup cooked chickpeas or 1 (15-ounce) can chickpeas, rinsed and drained
- 12 ounces fresh, canned, or thawed frozen artichoke hearts
- 1 pint cherry tomatoes, halved
- 1 cup thawed frozen shelled edamame
- ½ cup chopped fresh cilantro
- 1 cup chopped cremini mushrooms
- 4 ounces fresh mozzarella, diced

MAKE THE DRESSING:

In a small bowl combine all of the dressing ingredients except the oil and whisk until well mixed. Slowly pour in the oil while whisking constantly. Whisk until the dressing has thickened slightly.

ASSEMBLE THE SALAD:

Combine all of the salad ingredients in a medium bowl and toss until the greens and beans are evenly distributed. Spoon the dressing over the salad and give it a thorough toss until everything is well coated in dressing. Serve immediately. Leftover salad can be stored in the refrigerator for up to 3 days.

Nutritional analysis per serving (1 cup): calories 161, fat 1 g, saturated fat 1 g, cholesterol 7 mg, fiber 6 g, protein 9 g, carbohydrate 20 g, sodium 131 mg

ROASTED VEGGIE AND CHICKEN CHOPPED SALAD

The roasted chicken in this salad makes it hearty and savory. Cruciferous vegetables are wonderful to eat raw if you like some crunch. Lightly steam the cauliflower and broccoli if you prefer softer vegetables.

- ½ small head broccoli, cut into small florets
- ½ small head cauliflower, chopped
- 6 baby carrots, chopped
- 1 red bell pepper, seeded and chopped
- ½ medium red onion, finely chopped
- 1 garlic clove, minced
- 6 ounces chopped cooked chicken breast
- 2 tablespoons extra-virgin olive oil
- red pepper flakes
- sea salt and freshly ground black pepper to taste
- 2 tablespoon grated Parmigiano Reggiano cheese

Serves: 2

Prep time: 15 minutes

Level: Easy

Budget: $

Combine the vegetables and garlic in a medium bowl and toss until mixed well. Crumble the chicken over the vegetables and dress with the olive oil. Season to taste with red pepper flakes, salt, and black pepper and mix until all of the vegetables are seasoned. Sprinkle the cheese over the salad and serve.

Nutritional analysis per serving (1 cup): calories 249, fat 7 g, saturated fat 2 g, cholesterol 77 mg, fiber 6 g, protein 33 g, carbohydrate 14 g, sodium 707 mg

SOBA NOODLE SALAD WITH BOK CHOY

Soba noodles made of 100% buckwheat are a special gluten-free treat. Combined with bok choy and Asian dressing, this salad is a winner!

Serves: 12

Prep time:
20 minutes

Cook time:
25 minutes

Level: Easy

Budget: $

NOODLES:

- 2 (8-ounce) packages soba noodles
- 1 tablespoon sesame oil
- ¼ cup grapeseed oil
- ¼ cup chopped roasted unsalted almonds
- ¼ cup white sesame seeds
- 1 large bok choy, trimmed and thinly sliced
- ½ bunch (about 1 ½ ounces) fresh cilantro, roughly chopped
- 1 bunch (about 4 ounces) scallions, thinly sliced

DRESSING:

- ½ cup tahini paste
- ¼ cup almond butter
- ½ cup apple cider vinegar
- 2 tablespoons reduced-sodium, gluten-free tamari
- juice of 1 lime
- sea salt and freshly ground black pepper to taste
- ½ cup extra-virgin olive oil

MAKE THE NOODLES:

1. Heat a large pot of unsalted water over high heat until boiling. Reduce the heat to medium and wait until the water is at a brisk simmer. Add the soba noodles to the pot and stir gently so they don't stick.

2. Cook the noodles until just past al dente, 6–8 minutes. Drain the noodles and run cold water over them for 3–4 minutes to cool them down. Drain any excess water and transfer the noodles to a bowl. Toss them with the sesame oil to prevent sticking.

3. Heat the grapeseed oil in a medium cast-iron pan over medium-heat. Add the noodles, almonds, and sesame seeds and stir-fry until the nuts and seeds are toasted and the noodles are hot, 4–5 minutes.

4. Transfer the contents of the pan to a platter or large serving bowl, leaving any excess oil behind in the pan.

MAKE THE DRESSING:

Combine all of the dressing ingredients except the oil in a blender. Blend on medium speed while slowly pouring in the oil until smooth and emulsified.

ASSEMBLE THE SALAD:

Scatter the bok choy, cilantro, and scallions over the bed of noodles and dress only the amount you are going to serve immediately. Leave any leftover noodles undressed for storing. They will keep in the refrigerator for up to 3 days.

Nutritional analysis per serving (¾ cup): calories 417, fat 28 g, saturated fat 4 g, cholesterol 0 mg, fiber 4 g, protein 11 g, carbohydrate 33 g, sodium 364 mg

KRISTEN'S KALE WALDORF

Serves: 4

Prep time:
10 minutes

Level: Easy

Budget: $

If you love some crunch in your salad, this version of a Waldorf salad is for you. The apples and walnuts add not only interest to your palate but also loads of healthy anti–inflammatory nutrients.

DRESSING:

- 2 tablespoons apple cider vinegar
- 3 tablespoons extra-virgin olive oil
- sea salt and freshly ground black pepper

SALAD:

- 1 bunch Lacinato or black kale, stemmed and chopped
- 2 small apples, cored and chopped
- ⅓ cup chopped walnuts

MAKE THE DRESSING:

In a small bowl whisk the vinegar while slowly pouring in the olive oil. Season to taste with salt and black pepper.

ASSEMBLE THE SALAD:

In a medium bowl combine the kale, apples, and walnuts. Pour the dressing over the kale, toss until evenly coated, and serve.

Nutritional analysis per serving (1 cup): calories 238, fat 17 g, saturated fat 2 g, cholesterol 0 mg, fiber 5 g, protein 4 g, carbohydrate 23 g, sodium 31 mg

ENTRÉES

COCONUT-FLOUR FLATBREAD SANDWICH

Serves: 1

Prep time:
5 minutes

Cook time:
20 minutes

Level: Easy

Budget: $

Low-glycemic bread is possible when coconut flour is used, due to its high-fiber content. Use high-quality, organic Parmesan cheese to maximize flavor and health.

FLATBREAD:

- 1 large egg
- 1 tablespoon coconut flour
- 2 tablespoons whole milk
- ½ teaspoon pizza seasoning
- ¼ teaspoon garlic powder
- 1 tablespoon grated Parmigiano Reggiano cheese
- 2 teaspoons extra-virgin olive oil

FILLING:

- 4 cherry tomatoes, sliced
- 2 ounces fresh mozzarella, diced
- 4 fresh basil leaves, chopped
- sea salt and freshly ground black pepper to taste

1. In a medium bowl mix all of the flatbread ingredients except the oil, until the batter is smooth. Let rest for 5–10 minutes.

2. Heat 1 teaspoon of the oil in a large cast-iron pan over medium heat. When hot, pour half of the batter into the pan to form a 4- to 5-inch circle. Repeat with the remaining batter so you have two small circles.

3. Cook until the bottoms of the flatbreads are golden brown, 2–3 minutes. Flip the flatbreads and scatter the fillings over one of them. Cook until the bottoms are golden brown, 2 minutes.

4. Place the flatbread with no filling on top of the one with filling and reduce the heat to low. Remove the sandwich from the pan once the cheese has fully melted. Drizzle over the remaining 1 teaspoon oil and serve.

Nutritional analysis per serving (1 sandwich): calories 253, fat 19 g, saturated fat 11 g, cholesterol 202 mg, fiber 3 g, protein 10 g, carbohydrate 8 g, sodium 396 mg

CHUNKY AVOCADO TACOS

Avocados, cilantro, jalapeño, and lime create a spicy, delicious filling for the warm sprouted corn taco shells.

- 4 sprouted corn taco shells
- flesh of 2 avocados
- juice of 1 lime
- ½ small white onion, finely chopped
- 1 small tomato, finely chopped
- ½ small jalapeño pepper, seeded and finely chopped
- ¼ cup chopped fresh cilantro
- sea salt

Serves: 4

Prep time: 10 minutes

Cook time: 5 minutes

Level: Easy

Budget: $

1. Preheat the oven to 350°F.
2. Place the taco shells on a baking sheet or sheet tray and toast for 4–5 minutes. Let cool while you make the filling.
3. Place the avocado flesh in a medium bowl. Use a large fork or potato masher to mash the avocados until spreadable but still chunky.
4. Add the lime juice, onion, tomato, jalapeño, cilantro, and salt to taste and mix well. Taste for seasoning and add more salt or lime juice if desired.
5. Fill each shell with a few tablespoons of the avocado mixture and serve immediately.

Nutritional analysis per serving (1 taco): calories 239, fat 18 g, saturated fat 2 g, cholesterol 0 mg, fiber 8 g, protein 3 g, carbohydrate 19 g, sodium 11 mg

Latin Black Bean Burgers

Serves: 6

Prep time:
10 minutes

Cook time:
40 minutes

Level:
Moderate

Budget: $

This wonderful, simple bean burger incorporates oats as well as nuts and seeds to help balance your blood sugar. This recipe calls for gluten-free oats, which are tolerated by many but can still contain gluten. Try these burgers as you reintroduce gluten and see how you feel.

- ½ cup rolled gluten-free oats
- ¼ cup pumpkin seeds
- 2 medium carrots, peeled and grated
- 3 cups cooked black beans or 1½ (15-ounce) cans black beans, rinsed and drained
- ½ teaspoon ground cinnamon
- ½ teaspoon ground cumin
- ½ teaspoon ground coriander
- ½ teaspoon smoked paprika
- 2 tablespoons extra-virgin olive oil
- sea salt and freshly ground black pepper
- ½ cup fresh or thawed frozen corn
- 1 avocado, peeled, pitted, and sliced, for garnish

1. Preheat the oven to 300°F.
2. Put the oats and pumpkin seeds in a food processor and pulse until coarsely ground. Add the carrots, 2 cups of the beans, all of the spices, and the olive oil. Season to taste with salt and black pepper and pulse until the mixture is well blended.
3. Transfer the black bean mixture to a medium bowl and fold in the remaining 1 cup beans and the corn. Wet your hands and form 6 patties.
4. Place the patties on a nonstick baking sheet and bake, flipping once halfway through the cooking, until crisp, about 40 minutes.

5. Remove the burgers from the oven and transfer to a wire rack to cool. Garnish with the avocado and serve. Any leftover black bean mixture can be stored in the refrigerator for up to 4 days.

Nutritional analysis per serving (1 burger): calories 391, fat 12 g, saturated fat 2 g, cholesterol 0 mg, fiber 13 g, protein 19 g, carbohydrate 56 g, sodium 251 mg

HEARTY GREENS WITH GINGER AND SUGAR SNAP PEAS OVER SOBA

Serves: 5

Prep time: 15 minutes

Cook time: 30 minutes

Level: Easy

Budget: $

This light and refreshing meal explodes with flavor. You will love the aroma of sesame oil infused into the soba noodles.

- 1 (8-ounce) package soba noodles
- 1 tablespoon sesame oil
- 2 tablespoons extra-virgin coconut oil
- 1-inch piece fresh ginger, peeled and grated
- sea salt to taste
- 1 tablespoon mustard seeds
- 1 tablespoon cumin seeds
- 1 large bunch kale, stemmed and chopped
- 3 large rainbow chard leaves, stemmed and chopped
- 2 large mustard green leaves, stemmed and chopped
- 1 cup sugar snap peas, finely sliced
- ¼ cup chopped fresh cilantro
- 1 teaspoon white sesame seeds

1. Heat a large pot of unsalted water over high heat. When it boils, reduce the heat to medium and wait until the water is at a brisk simmer. Add the soba noodles to the pot and stir gently so they don't stick.

2. Cook the noodles until just past al dente, 6–8 minutes. Drain the noodles and run cold water over them for 3–4 minutes to cool them down. Drain any excess water and transfer the noodles to a bowl. Toss them with the sesame oil to prevent sticking.

3. Heat the coconut oil in a medium cast-iron pan over medium heat. After a minute add the ginger, salt, mustard seeds, and cumin seeds. Stir-fry the spices until the mustard seeds are popping and toasted, about 2 minutes.

4. Add the greens and toss them until coated in the ginger and spices. Cook the greens until wilted and tender, 3–4 minutes.

5. Pour the contents of the pan over the soba noodles. Garnish the greens with the sugar snap peas, cilantro, and sesame seeds. Serve immediately. Store any leftovers in a glass container in your refrigerator. Discard after 3 days.

Nutritional analysis per serving (¾ cup): calories 157, fat 5 g, saturated fat 3 g, cholesterol 0 mg, fiber 3 g, protein 4 g, carbohydrate 25 g, sodium 20 mg

SPICY BLACK BEAN BURGERS

Serves: 4

Prep time:
15 minutes

Cook time:
15 minutes

Level:
Moderate

Budget: $

Black beans are rich in anthocyanins as well as short-chain fatty acids, which feed the healthy bacteria in the lower digestive tract. This makes for a wonderful vegetarian meal, filled with savory spices to perk up your palate.

- 2 tablespoons extra-virgin olive oil
- 1 teaspoon ground cumin
- ½ teaspoon ground turmeric
- ¼ teaspoon cayenne pepper
- 1 small Vidalia onion, finely chopped
- 1 medium red bell pepper, seeded and finely chopped
- 4 garlic cloves, minced
- 1½ cups cooked black beans or 1 (15-ounce) can black beans, rinsed and drained
- 1½ cups cooked brown rice
- 2 cups almond meal
- sea salt and freshly ground black pepper
- 1 lime, cut into wedges
- hot pepper sauce (optional)

1. Heat 1 tablespoon of the oil in a medium cast-iron pan over medium-high heat.
2. Add the spices and toast them for 30 seconds. Lower the heat to medium and toss in the onion, bell pepper, and garlic and cook the vegetables in the spices until the onions are translucent, 5–7 minutes.
3. Turn off the heat and transfer the cooked vegetables to a food processor. Pulse until almost puréed.
4. Add the beans, rice, and almond meal to the food processor, season to taste with salt and black pepper, and pulse until the beans are mostly puréed and the almond meal is distributed evenly.
5. Wet your hands and form the bean mixture into 4 patties.

6. Heat the remaining 1 tablespoon oil in a large cast-iron pan. When hot, lay the burgers in the pan. Cook until lightly golden brown, 3–5 minutes per side. Remove from the pan and cool briefly on a wire rack.

7. Serve with lime wedges and hot sauce, if desired. Any uncooked black bean mixture can be stored in the refrigerator for up to 4 days.

Nutritional analysis per serving (1 burger): calories 522, fat 32 g, saturated fat 8 g, cholesterol 0 mg, fiber 13 g, protein 18 g, carbohydrate 46 g, sodium 164 mg

NUTTY SALMON SALAD

Serves: 4

Prep time:
5 minutes

Level: Easy

Budget: $

This salad is loaded with anti-inflammatory nutrients. Omega-3 fats from the salmon, ellagic acid from the walnuts, and curcumin from the turmeric transform a traditional "tuna" salad into a Blood Sugar Solution version for a healthy, sustainable meal.

DRESSING:

- ¼ teaspoon curry powder
- ⅛ teaspoon ground turmeric
- 1 tablespoon mayonnaise
- juice of ½ lemon
- sea salt and freshly ground black pepper to taste

SALAD:

- 2 (12-ounce) cans wild salmon, drained
- 1 tablespoon finely chopped red onion
- 1 tablespoon finely chopped celery
- ½ medium apple, finely chopped
- 8 walnuts, chopped

MAKE THE DRESSING:

In a small bowl combine all of the dressing ingredients and whisk until thickened and emulsified.

ASSEMBLE THE SALAD:

Combine all of the salad ingredients in a medium bowl and toss until evenly mixed. Spoon the dressing over the salad and mix until everything is well coated. Serve immediately. Any leftover salad can be refrigerated for up to 2 days.

Nutritional analysis per serving (¾ cup): calories 143, fat 4 g, saturated fat 3 g, cholesterol 40 mg, fiber 1 g, protein 23 g, carbohydrate 3 g, sodium 568 mg

ROASTED APPLE AND SWEET POTATO MEDLEY

Using chicken sausage is a convenient and quick way to add lean protein and complexity to a simple medley of roasted vegetables. The sage adds warmth and earthy body to the dish. The avocado provides a smooth texture and healthy monounsaturated fat as well.

Serves: 6

Prep time: 5 minutes

Cook time: 40 minutes

Level: Easy

Budget: $

- 2 medium sweet potatoes, cut into 1-inch cubes
- 2 medium red potatoes, cut into 1-inch cubes
- 6 sweet baby peppers, stemmed and halved (or 2 bell peppers, seeded and cut into quarters)
- 1 medium apple, peeled, cored, and cut into 1-inch cubes
- 3 tablespoons extra-virgin olive oil
- 2 tablespoons dried sage
- 1 tablespoon dried thyme
- sea salt and freshly ground black pepper to taste
- 1 (12-ounce) package chicken sausage, thinly sliced
- 1 medium yellow onion, thinly sliced
- 3 garlic cloves, minced
- 1 avocado, peeled, pitted, and chopped

1. Preheat the oven to 400°F.
2. In a large bowl toss the potatoes, peppers, and apple in 2 tablespoons of the oil and season with the sage, thyme, salt, and black pepper. Transfer to a roasting pan and spread out in a single layer. Roast for 30 minutes, stirring occasionally.
3. While the vegetables roast, heat a large cast-iron pan over medium heat and add the remaining 1 tablespoon oil. Put the sausage in the pan and cook until brown on all sides, 3–5 minutes.
4. Add the onion and garlic and season to taste with salt and black pepper. Stir until well coated in the sausage juices and cook until caramelized and soft, 7–8 minutes. Turn off the heat and transfer the sausage mixture to a large platter.

5. Transfer the roasted vegetables to the platter of sausage and garnish with the chopped avocado. Leftover sausage can be refrigerated for up to 3 days.

Nutritional analysis per serving (1½ cups): calories 340, fat 14 g, saturated fat 2 g, cholesterol 32 mg, fiber 10 g, protein 14 g, carbohydrate 42 g, sodium 182 mg

CHICKEN SALVATORE

The key to making this tasty stir-fry is to not overcook the chicken breasts. Properly cooked chicken yields a juicy meal accented by the sautéed vegetables.

- ¼ cup extra-virgin olive oil
- 6 garlic cloves, minced
- 1 cup cremini mushrooms, thinly sliced
- 1 large red onion, thinly sliced
- 4 (4-ounce) boneless, skinless chicken breasts, cut into bite-size pieces
- 1 medium red bell pepper, seeded and thinly sliced
- 1 medium yellow bell pepper, seeded and thinly sliced
- 1½ cups cooked brown rice
- sea salt and freshly ground black pepper
- 1 large tomato, diced
- ½ cup grated Parmigiano Reggiano cheese
- ½ cup grated pecorino cheese
- ¼ cup chopped fresh parsley

Serves: 6

Prep time: 20 minutes

Cook time: 20 minutes

Level: Easy

Budget: $

1. Heat the oil in a large sauté pan over medium-high heat. Once the oil is hot add the garlic, mushrooms, and onion. Cook, stirring frequently, until the vegetables are soft, 6–7 minutes.

2. Add the chicken and bell peppers and stir-fry until the chicken is cooked and golden brown, 4–5 minutes.

3. Reduce the heat to low and add the brown rice. Toss the rice with the vegetable and chicken mixture until coated and warmed through. Season to taste with salt and black pepper and toss until well mixed.

4. Transfer to a serving dish and garnish with the tomato, cheese, and parsley. Serve while hot. Any leftover chicken can be refrigerated for up to 3 days.

Nutritional analysis per serving (1 cup): calories 527, fat 23 g, saturated fat 6 g, cholesterol 111 mg, fiber 5 g, protein 48 g, carbohydrate 35 g, sodium 698 mg

ALMOND-CRUSTED CHICKEN BREASTS

Serves: 4

Prep time:
15 minutes

Cook time:
40 minutes

Level: Easy

Budget: $

This chicken is encrusted with basil-infused almond meal instead of bread-crumbs. The texture adds crunch without the gluten.

- 1 cup roasted almonds
- 1 cup grated Parmigiano Reggiano cheese
- 1 teaspoon dried basil
- ¼ cup fresh basil leaves
- sea salt and freshly ground black pepper
- 2 (8-ounce) boneless, skinless chicken breasts
- 2 tablespoons extra-virgin olive oil
- 1 lemon, cut into wedges

1. Preheat the oven to 400°F.
2. Grind the almonds in a food processor until they are close to the consistency of breadcrumbs. Add the cheese and dried and fresh basil, reserving 4 leaves of the fresh basil for garnishing, and season the mixture to taste with salt and black pepper. Pulse the mixture until the basil is finely chopped and evenly distributed throughout.
3. Pound the chicken breasts between two pieces of plastic wrap with a large mallet or the bottom of a heavy pan, until each breast is ¾ inch thick.
4. Season the chicken on both sides with salt and black pepper.
5. Pour the almond crumbs onto a large plate and firmly press the chicken pieces into them, coating both sides.
6. Grease the bottom of a broiler pan with 1 tablespoon of the oil and add the chicken breasts to the pan. Drizzle the remaining 1 table-spoon oil evenly over the chicken and slide the pan into the oven on the top rack.

7. Bake until the crust is golden brown and the chicken is cooked through, 20–25 minutes. Transfer the chicken to a platter. Serve with lemon wedges and garnish with the reserved fresh basil leafs.

Nutritional analysis per serving (½ chicken breast): calories 352, fat 24 g, saturated fat 5 g, cholesterol 58 mg, fiber 4 g, protein 28 g, carbohydrate 7 g, sodium 450 mg

RASPBERRY PISTACHIO-CRUSTED CHICKEN WITH STEAMED KALE AND WILD RICE

Serves: 4

Prep time: 15 minutes

Cook time: 55 minutes

Level: Easy

Budget: $

Sweet and nutty, with a combination of raspberries and pistachios, this dinner can dress up an evening or create a delicious treat for the family.

- 1 cup fresh or thawed frozen raspberries
- 1 tablespoon Dijon mustard
- juice of ½ large lemon
- ½ cup uncooked wild rice
- 1½ cups water
- sea salt to taste
- 2 (8-ounce) boneless, skinless chicken breasts, halved crosswise
- ½ cup whole-grain breadcrumbs
- 2 tablespoons chopped pistachio nuts
- 2 tablespoons chopped fresh parsley
- freshly ground white pepper to taste
- 1 tablespoon plus 1 teaspoon extra-virgin olive oil
- 2 garlic cloves, minced
- 1 large bunch kale, stemmed and cut into 3-inch pieces

1. Combine the raspberries, mustard, and lemon juice in a small food processor or blender and blend until smooth. Transfer to a large bowl.

2. Put the wild rice, water, and a pinch of salt in a medium saucepan and bring to a boil. When it boils, reduce the heat to low, cover, and simmer until the liquid has evaporated and the rice is tender, 50–55 minutes.

3. Place the chicken breasts between two sheets of plastic wrap and pound them with a kitchen mallet until they are ½ inch thick.

4. Add the chicken breasts to the bowl with the raspberry sauce and toss the pieces until evenly coated in the sauce.

5. Combine the breadcrumbs, pistachios, parsley, salt, and pepper on a large plate and gently press the chicken into the mixture until evenly coated on both sides.

6. Heat 1 tablespoon of the oil in a large cast-iron pan over medium-high heat. Cook the chicken until the crust is golden brown and crisp, 3–5 minutes per side. Transfer the chicken to a platter to rest.

7. Put the pan back over medium heat and add the remaining 1 teaspoon oil and the garlic. Add the kale to the pan and season it to taste with salt and white pepper. Cook the kale until it wilts, 4–5 minutes.

8. Serve the chicken on top of the wild rice with the kale on the side. Any leftover chicken can be refrigerated for up to 3 days.

Nutritional analysis per serving (1 breast, 1 cup kale, ⅓ cup rice): calories 436, fat 11 g, saturated fat 2 g, cholesterol 66 mg, fiber 11 g, protein 41 g, carbohydrate 48 g, sodium 420 mg

CRANBERRY TURKEY WRAP

Serves: 2

Prep time:
15 minutes

Level: Easy

Budget: $

Look for natural cranberry relish that does not contain high-fructose corn syrup, as this is a delicious addition to poultry dishes and a nutritious condiment to replace mayonnaise. BroccoSprouts contain loads of cancer-fighting phytonutrients called glucosinolates, and they add a flavorful zip to any sandwich, wrap, or salad.

- ¼ cup whole cranberry relish
- 2 sprouted-grain tortillas
- 6 ounces roast turkey breast, sliced
- 1 medium avocado, peeled, pitted, and sliced
- 1 small pickling cucumber, sliced
- ½ cup broccoli sprouts or other sprouts

Spread the cranberry relish over the tortillas. Line the middle of each tortilla with half of the turkey, avocado, cucumber, and sprouts. Roll tightly into a burrito shape and serve.

Nutritional analysis per serving (1 wrap): calories 465, fat 18 g, saturated fat 0 g, cholesterol 43 mg, fiber 13 g, protein 26 g, carbohydrate 55 g, sodium 290 mg

MEXICAN LASAGNA

An artful display of bright colors from the various layers in this Mexican version of lasagna makes this an irresistible dish. Use organic cheese to ensure the ultimate in quality and health value.

- 2 tablespoon extra-virgin olive oil
- 1½ pounds lean ground turkey
- sea salt
- 6 gluten-free sprouted corn tortillas
- 2 (16-ounce) cans refried beans
- ½ cup Oaxaca or mozzarella cheese, grated
- hot pepper sauce to taste
- ¼ cup sour cream
- ½ large white onion, chopped
- 1 large tomato, roughly chopped
- 3 tablespoons chopped fresh cilantro
- juice of 1 lime
- 1 lime, cut into wedges

Serves: 6

Prep time: 15 minutes

Cook time: 25 minutes

Level: Easy

Budget: $

1. Preheat the oven to 325°F.
2. Heat the oil in a wide cast-iron pan over medium-high heat. Add the turkey, season it to taste with salt, and break it up as it cooks. Cook the turkey until brown, 6–8 minutes. Transfer to a plate and reserve.
3. Turn off the heat and place two tortillas in the bottom of the pan so the edges overlap by 2 inches.
4. Spread half of the beans across the tortillas and sprinkle over half of the cheese.
5. Add two more tortillas on top and cover with the browned turkey. Add a few shakes of hot pepper sauce (or more if you like it hot) to the turkey and cover with another layer of tortilla. Top with the remaining beans and cheese and put the pan in the oven.
6. Bake until the cheese is melted and the beans are heated through, 15–20 minutes.

7. Remove the pan from the oven and transfer the lasagna to a platter. Garnish with a few tablespoons of sour cream and sprinkle on the onion, tomatoes, and cilantro. Drizzle the lime juice across the top of the lasagna and serve with extra lime wedges on the side. Serve immediately.

Nutritional analysis per serving (⅙ lasagna): calories 490, fat 18 g, saturated fat 5 g, cholesterol 82 mg, fiber 12 g, protein 34 g, carbohydrate 51 g, sodium 800 mg

BLUE CHEESE COWBOY BURGER

A traditional burger with tangy blue cheese. Use grass-fed lean beef to elevate the omega-3 content in this burger and benefit from disease-fighting conjugated linoleic acid (CLA), which is found only in grass-fed beef and certain kinds of dairy like blue cheese.

- 1 pound grass-fed lean ground beef
- sea salt and freshly ground black pepper
- 1 tablespoon unsalted butter
- 1 tablespoon grapeseed oil
- 1 small Vidalia onion, finely chopped
- ⅓ cup blue cheese, crumbled

Serves: 4

Prep time: 5 minutes

Cook time: 10 minutes

Level: Easy

Budget: $

1. Remove the beef from the refrigerator 30 minutes prior to cooking so it will cook more evenly.

2. Divide the beef into 4 equal sections and gently shape into patties. The more you compress and manipulate the meat, the grainier the texture will be once it cooks. Season both sides to taste with salt and black pepper. Gently press the seasonings into the meat with the palm of your hand.

3. Heat the butter and oil in a large cast-iron pan over medium heat. After two minutes lay the burgers in the pan and start to brown them. The key to a great burger is the crust; to get a good crust you have to let the beef sit undisturbed for at least 3–4 minutes.

4. After 3–4 minutes, carefully lift up one of the patties with a spatula to check how brown it is; you want a deep golden brown, not burnt meat. Lower the heat and take the burgers out of the pan briefly if they are browning too fast.

5. When you think they're ready to flip, add the onion to the pan in four little piles. Flip the burgers onto the onion piles and cook on top of the onions.

6. Add the blue cheese now if you want it melted over the tops of the burgers, otherwise just add it after the burger is cooked.

7. Cook until the onions are caramelized and the patties are cooked through, 3–4 minutes. Turn off the heat, transfer the burgers to a plate, and let rest for 3–4 minutes. Serve with your choice of condiments or with a lettuce "bun."

Nutritional analysis per serving (1 burger): calories 228, fat 5 g, saturated fat 8 g, cholesterol 0 mg, fiber 6 g, protein 7 g, carbohydrate 39 g, sodium 181 mg

SNACKS AND SIDES

BRAZIL NUT BARS

Nutty, slightly chewy, and lightly crunchy, these bars are a real powerhouse for sustaining energy.

- 1 tablespoon grapeseed oil
- 1½ cups raw Brazil nuts
- ½ cup raw pumpkin seeds
- ½ cup sliced toasted almonds
- ½ cup raw sunflower seeds
- ½ cup ground flaxseeds
- ⅓ cup dried cranberries
- 1 teaspoon ground cinnamon
- 2 cups gluten-free crispy brown-rice cereal
- 1 cup cashew butter
- ¾ cup honey

Serves: 16

Prep time: 15 minutes

Cook time: 3 minutes

Chill time: 30 minutes

Level: Easy

Budget: $

1. Lightly coat a 9 x 13-inch baking dish with grapeseed oil. Set aside.

2. Place the Brazil nuts in a food processor and pulse until the nuts are ground into a fine powder. Transfer to a large mixing bowl. Add the pumpkin seeds, almonds, sunflower seeds, flaxseeds, cranberries, cinnamon, and brown-rice cereal to the bowl.

3. Heat the cashew butter in a large saucepan over low heat. Add the honey and stir until very hot and bubbling, 2–3 minutes. Pour into the large mixing bowl and stir using a wooden spoon.

4. While the mixture is hot, press it firmly into the greased baking dish with a large spatula so it forms an even layer. Let the mixture cool in the refrigerator.

5. When cool, cut into 16 equal bars. The bars will keep for up to 4 months if stored in the freezer; wrap each bar individually with wax paper and defrost when ready to enjoy.

Nutritional analysis per serving (1 bar): calories 377, fat 27 g, saturated fat 5 g, cholesterol 0 mg, fiber 5 g, protein 10 g, carbohydrate 30 g, sodium 25 mg

Guilt-Free Cauliflower Pizza Bites

Cauliflower can become deliciously creamy when blended well. Make sure the cauliflower is dry before grating to ensure a creamy texture. These festive little bites are sure to please the palates of all family members, especially the younger ones. Choose a flavorful tomato sauce to accentuate that pizza-like feel.

Serves: 12

Prep time: 15 minutes

Cook time: 40 minutes

Level: Easy

Budget: $

- 3 tablespoons extra-virgin olive oil
- 1½ cups cauliflower florets
- sea salt and freshly ground black pepper
- 2 large egg whites
- 1 cup 1% milk-fat cottage cheese, drained
- 2 teaspoons dried parsley
- 1 teaspoon dried oregano
- ½ teaspoon garlic powder
- 2 cups spicy marinara sauce
- 4 fresh basil leaves, finely sliced
- 6 fresh oregano leaves, chopped

1. Preheat the oven to 450°F. Line a mini muffin pan with 12 baking cups and lightly grease the cups with 1 teaspoon of the oil. Set aside.

2. Grate the cauliflower using the shredder disc attachment on a food processor. The pieces should be approximately the size of uncooked rice grains.

3. Heat a large cast-iron pan over medium–high heat and add 2 tablespoons of the oil. Add the cauliflower, season to taste with salt and black pepper, and cook until slightly translucent, 6–8 minutes. Transfer to a large, wide bowl and let cool.

4. Place the egg whites, cottage cheese, parsley, oregano, and garlic powder in a food processor and season to taste with salt and black pepper. Blend until smooth.

5. Add the blended ingredients to the bowl with the cooked cauliflower and mix thoroughly.

6. Spoon an equal amount of the mixture into each baking cup, packing the mixture down into the corners of each cup as you fill them.

7. Brush the tops with the remaining 2 teaspoons oil and bake until golden brown, 25–30 minutes.

8. Remove the pizza bites from the oven and let them cool completely in the pan; this will ensure they hold when taken out of the muffin cups (they are quite fragile when hot).

9. While the pizza bites cool, warm the tomato sauce in a small saucepan over low heat. Garnish the bites with the fresh basil and oregano and serve with the warm tomato sauce on the side for dipping. Leftover bites can be stored in the refrigerator for up to 3 days.

Nutritional analysis per serving (1 pizza bite): calories 34, fat 2 g, saturated fat 1 g, cholesterol 2 mg, fiber 1 g, protein 4 g, carbohydrate 2 g, sodium 90 mg

FIVE TASTE SENSES IN ONE PERFECT BITE

This appetizer is simple to make yet tantalizes the senses with its complex flavors and textures. It is the epitome of the perfect bite—encompassing all five taste senses of sweet, salty, bitter, sour, and umami in one mouth-watering bite.

- ½ small watermelon
- 4 ounces goat cheese, at room temperature
- 10 kalamata olives, pitted and halved
- ½ cup fresh basil, finely sliced
- 1 tablespoon extra-virgin olive oil

Serves: 10

Prep time: 15 minutes

Level: Easy

Budget: $

1. Remove the rind from the watermelon and cut it into rectangular blocks that are about 2 x 5 inches.

2. Lay the pieces flat on a cutting board and spread a thin layer of goat cheese on each piece.

3. Place two olive halves, cut sides down, on the cheese, scatter fresh basil on top, and drizzle lightly with olive oil. Serve chilled or at room temperature.

Nutritional analysis per serving (1 piece): calories 84, fat 5 g, saturated fat 2 g, cholesterol 9 mg, fiber 1 g, protein 3 g, carbohydrate 7 g, sodium 150 mg

DANDELION DIP

Serves: 6

Prep time:
5 minutes

Cook time:
15 minutes

Chill time:
1 hour

Level: Easy

Budget: $

Dandelion greens are an excellent and underrated wild green with powerful detoxification properties. The nutty flavor and creamy texture of the tahini are a wonderful balance to the slightly bitter taste of the greens.

- sea salt
- 1 large bunch dandelion greens, finely chopped
- 3 tablespoons extra-virgin olive oil
- ¾ cup full-fat plain Greek yogurt
- ¼ cup tahini
- juice of ½ lemon

1. Fill a large pot with water and bring to a boil over high heat.
2. Add a large pinch of salt and add the greens to the pot. Boil until completely tender, about 15 minutes. Drain.
3. Put the cooked greens into a food processor and add the remaining ingredients. Pulse until the mixture is smooth and blended. Check for seasoning and add more salt or lemon juice to taste.
4. Chill in the refrigerator for at least 1 hour. Serve as a dip alongside gluten-free crackers or raw vegetables. Leftover dip can be refrigerated for up to 4 days.

Nutritional analysis per serving (¾ cup): calories 91, fat 6 g, saturated fat 1 g, cholesterol 2 mg, fiber 2 g, protein 4 g, carbohydrate 6 g, sodium 203 mg

7

Desserts

While on the Blood Sugar Solution I encourage you to eliminate all sugar from your diet—from syrup to soda. (Once in a while having some high-quality dark chocolate—70 percent dark cacao—is fine and even encouraged.) When you begin to transition off the program, I want you to see that the Blood Sugar Solution is actually a lifelong investment in your health and vitality. If you eat according to the guidelines in my book 90 percent of the time, there's 10 percent wiggle room for savory or sweet treats. The following are doctor-approved options to have in moderation. The most important advice I can give you is this: stay present in the act of enjoying your treats when you have them. Savor them in small amounts. After all, birthdays, weddings, anniversaries, graduations, holidays, and rituals are the traditions that make life truly sweet! I want you to eat to live, not the other way around. If you know you don't tolerate sugar or gluten well or that certain foods trigger you to overeat, stay away from them. Otherwise, take pleasure in these creative, anti-inflammatory desserts without the toxic hangover of the white menace (white sugar, white flour, and white rice).

PINK POM POM

Serves: 2

Prep time:
5 minutes

Level: Easy

Budget: $

Between the maca root (a South American superfood), pomegranate, berries, and coconut oil, this is one spectacular super-dessert. Enjoy it when you crave a sweet yet healthy and refreshing drink. Pomegranate powder is also a super-food, made from dried pomegranates, which have potent phytochemicals and add a slightly sweet, satisfying taste.

- 2 tablespoons pomegranate powder
- 1 cup frozen mixed berries
- 2 cups unsweetened almond milk
- 1 teaspoon pure vanilla extract
- 1 tablespoon extra-virgin coconut oil
- 1 tablespoon maca powder

Combine all of the ingredients in a blender and blend on high speed until smooth, 1–2 minutes. If the smoothie is too thick, thin it with a little more almond milk or water; it should be thick but drinkable. Serve immediately.

Nutritional analysis per serving (1 cup): calories 188, fat 3 g, saturated fat 6 g, cholesterol 0 mg, fiber 3 g, protein 2 g, carbohydrate 23 g, sodium 216 mg

GUILT-FREE CHOCOLATE MOUSSE

The secret to this dessert lies in choosing the right avocado. Look for an avocado that is ripe and slightly malleable to the touch. This mousse also has the magic of cocoa, which delights your taste buds and your metabolism.

- flesh of 1 avocado
- 1 tablespoon pure maple syrup
- ¼ cup unsweetened cocoa powder
- ½ large banana
- 2 tablespoons water
- 2 teaspoons pure vanilla extract
- 1 tablespoon strong brewed decaf coffee
- sea salt to taste
- 1 pint fresh raspberries (optional)

Serves: 4

Prep time: 5 minutes

Level: Easy

Budget: $

Combine all of the ingredients in a blender and blend on medium speed until smooth and creamy, 1–2 minutes. If the mousse is too thick, thin it with a little extra coffee or water. It should similar to the consistency of pudding but slightly lighter. Serve immediately. Leftover mousse can be refrigerated for up to 5 days.

Nutritional analysis per serving (½ cup): calories 124, fat 8 g, saturated fat 2 g, cholesterol 9 mg, fiber 5 g, protein 2 g, carbohydrate 14 g, sodium 43 mg

Dark Chocolate Silk Pudding

Serves: 2

Prep time:
10 minutes

Level: Easy

Budget: $

Raw, organic cacao adds richness to this pudding as well as potent antioxidants, sulfur, and magnesium. Cacao comes from the bean of the cacao fruit, which is dried into a powder at low temperatures to preserve the flavor and quality. Goji berries come from Asia, are bright red, and supply a plethora of healing antioxidants, which have been shown to prevent and reverse chronic disease. You can find them in your local natural foods store.

- ½ cup fresh blueberries
- 1 tablespoon honey
- 1 tablespoon pure vanilla extract
- 3 tablespoons coconut water
- 2 tablespoons plus 1 teaspoon cacao powder
- flesh of 1 avocado
- sea salt to taste
- 6 goji berries (optional)
- 2 teaspoons matcha green tea powder (optional)

1. Combine the blueberries, honey, vanilla, and 2 tablespoons of the coconut water in a blender and blend on medium speed until smooth.

2. Turn the blender down to low and gradually add the cocoa powder until evenly mixed. Add the avocado, remaining 1 tablespoon coconut water, and salt and blend until incorporated.

3. If the pudding is too thick, add more coconut water until it is smooth but slightly stiff. Serve chilled, garnished with a few goji berries and a spoonful of green tea powder sprinkled on top. Any leftover pudding can be stored in the refrigerator for up to 5 days.

Nutritional analysis per serving (½ cup): calories 200, fat 11 g, saturated fat 2 g, cholesterol 0 mg, fiber 8 g, protein 3 g, carbohydrate 23 g, sodium 28 mg

FROZEN FUN POPS

Rhubarb is a wonderful vegetable that lowers the glycemic load of any meal. Combined with berries and chocolate, it creates a wonderful, sweet frozen dessert.

- 1 tablespoon extra-virgin olive oil
- 1 pound fresh or frozen rhubarb, cut into ½-inch pieces
- 2 cups water
- 12 ounces frozen blueberries
- 2 ounces unsweetened chocolate, roughly chopped
- 4 ounces 70% dark chocolate, roughly chopped

Serves: 4

Prep time: 5 minutes

Cook time: 35 minutes

Chill time: 4–12 hours

Level: Easy

Budget: $

1. Heat the oil in a large sauté pan over medium heat. Add the rhubarb and pour in the water. Bring to a boil and cover the pan.

2. Reduce the heat to low and cook until the rhubarb is soft, about 15 minutes.

3. Add the blueberries and cook, stirring frequently, until the water is reduced by half, 10–12 minutes.

4. Stir in half of the unsweetened chocolate until evenly melted and cook the mixture down until it's the consistency of pudding, about 10 minutes.

5. Remove from the heat and let cool for 5 minutes in the pan. Fold in the rest of the chocolate pieces and pour the mixture into four 4-ounce freezer pop molds. Freeze overnight. You can also cover and refrigerate the mixture for 4 hours and serve it as pudding. Store any leftovers in the refrigerator for up to 3 days or in the freezer for up to 6 months.

Nutritional analysis per serving (one 4-ounce pop): calories 148, fat 7 g, saturated fat 3 g, cholesterol 0 mg, fiber 9 g, protein 4 g, carbohydrate 24 g, sodium 12 mg

STRAWBERRY ICE CREAM

Serves: 3

Prep time:
5 minutes

Chill time:
5 hours

Level: Easy

Budget: $

In this version of ice cream, the coconut provides unique health properties unseen in dairy-based versions, mostly from the medium-chain triglycerides and lauric acid. Lauric acid has been shown to have potent antimicrobial and antiparasitic properties that boost the immune system. Not only is this healthier than ice cream, but it has phenomenal texture and mouth-feel that mimics the famous creaminess we adore in traditional ice cream.

- 6 ounces unsweetened coconut milk
- 2 tablespoons extra-virgin coconut oil
- 1 teaspoon pure vanilla extract
- 12 large frozen strawberries

1. Chill the freezer bowl of an ice cream maker in the freezer for at least 2 hours before making the ice cream.

2. Combine all of the ingredients in a blender and blend on high speed until the strawberries are fully broken down and the mixture is creamy, 1–2 minutes. Transfer to the chilled ice cream bowl and start the machine. When churned, place the ice cream in the freezer until firm, 2–3 hours. The ice cream will keep for up to 6 months in the freezer.

Nutritional analysis per serving (½ cup): calories 228, fat 23 g, saturated fat 20 g, cholesterol 0 mg, fiber 2 g, protein 2 g, carbohydrate 7 g, sodium 9 mg

DOUBLE PEANUT BUTTER CHOCOLATE CUPS

Fun, flavorful, and packed with healthy fats from the coconut and peanuts, these homemade treats are an upgrade from the hydrogenated versions you should avoid at the store. You can substitute other nut butters or sunflower seed butter, but you'll need to adjust the honey to taste.

Serves: 10

Prep time: 15 minutes

Chill time: 30 minutes

Level: Easy

Budget: $

BOTTOM LAYER:

- 2 tablespoons extra-virgin coconut oil
- ¼ cup smooth peanut butter
- ½ teaspoon pure vanilla extract
- 2 tablespoons honey

TOP LAYER:

- 2 tablespoons extra-virgin coconut oil
- ¼ cup smooth peanut butter
- ¼ cup unsweetened cocoa powder
- ½ teaspoon pure vanilla extract
- 2 tablespoons honey

MAKE THE BOTTOM LAYER:

1. Combine all of the ingredients in a small bowl and mix until very smooth.

2. Set 10 mini baking cups in a mini muffin pan. Pour about one tablespoon of the bottom-layer mixture into each baking cup without dribbling it down the inside of the paper (or you'll get streaks in the final product). Place on a flat surface in the freezer.

MAKE THE TOP LAYER:

1. Combine all of the ingredients in a small bowl and mix until evenly incorporated. Remove the pan from the freezer and fill each baking cup to the top with the top-layer chocolate mixture.

2. Put the tray back in the freezer and let chill until the chocolate layer has hardened, about 15 minutes. Store the peanut butter cups in the freezer for up to 4 months.

Nutritional analysis per serving (1 peanut butter cup): calories 144, fat 13 g, saturated fat 7 g, cholesterol 0 mg, fiber 1 g, protein 4 g, carbohydrate 8 g, sodium 2 mg

DARK CHOCOLATE ALMOND-BUTTER BARK

Select raw almonds to preserve the healthy monounsaturated fats from oxidation. These treats are rich in phosphorous, magnesium, and calcium, all of which help you maintain healthy bones, while the fiber helps satiate you. The crunch in this bark separates it from other chocolate treats.

- 1 cup raw almonds
- 2 teaspoons extra-virgin coconut oil
- ½ teaspoon sea salt
- 7 ounces 70% dark chocolate, roughly chopped

Serves: 6

Prep time: 25 minutes

Chill time: 45 minutes

Level: Easy

Budget: $

1. Preheat the oven to 350°F.
2. Toast the almonds on a small baking sheet or sheet tray until golden brown, 5–8 minutes. Let cool.
3. Transfer the toasted almonds to a food processor. Add the coconut oil and salt and pulse until the mixture is the consistency of almond butter. Set aside.
4. Fill the bottom section of a double boiler with water and put it over low heat. Once hot, add the chocolate to the top section of the double boiler and place it over the bottom section. When all of the chocolate has melted, carefully pour half of it out onto a wax paper–lined baking sheet. Leave the remaining chocolate mixture in the double boiler and turn the heat down as low as possible.
5. Spread the chocolate on the wax paper into a ¼-inch-thick rectangle (about 10 x 6 inches) and put the baking sheet in the freezer. Let it harden for 15 minutes.
6. Remove the chocolate from the freezer and spread the toasted almond butter mixture across the surface of the chocolate. Leave a 1-inch border of chocolate around the edges.
7. Pour the remaining warm, melted chocolate over the almond butter and spread it to seal in the almond butter—around the edges you

should have chocolate on top of chocolate and in the center you should have almond butter between two layers of chocolate.

8. Put the baking sheet back in the freezer. After 30–40 minutes, remove the almond bark and cut it into 6 equal squares. Store the almond bark in the freezer for up to 4 months.

Nutritional analysis per serving (1 square): calories 183, fat 16 g, saturated fat 6 g, cholesterol 0 mg, fiber 4 g, protein 4 g, carbohydrate 9 g, sodium 42 mg

CHOCOLATE NUT CAKE

Serves: 6

Prep time:
5 minutes

Chill time:
30 minutes

Level: Easy

Budget: $

This cake is fast and easy to make and doesn't even require an oven. It is dense, velvety, and luscious from the coconut and almond butters. Blend the ingredients well for the smoothest texture. Coconut butter is made from coconut oil. It is rich in healthy saturated fats and has a subtle hint of natural sweetness. Find it in your local natural foods market.

- 10 pitted dates
- ¼ cup unsweetened cocoa powder
- ¼ cup plus 2 tablespoons coconut butter
- ¼ cup almond butter
- 1 tablespoon pure maple syrup
- 1 teaspoon pure vanilla extract
- ¼ teaspoon sea salt

1. Combine all of the ingredients in a food processor and blend until as smooth as possible, 3–5 minutes.
2. Spread the mixture into a greased mini loaf pan. Put the cake in the freezer for 30 minutes. When cold, slice into 6 pieces.

Nutritional analysis per serving (1 slice): calories 200, fat 15 g, saturated fat 8 g, cholesterol 82 mg, fiber 3 g, protein 6 g, carbohydrate 18 g, sodium 44 mg

LISA'S LEMON VANILLA CUPCAKES

Serves: 20

Prep time:
15 minutes

Cook time:
30 minutes

Level: Easy

Budget: $

Low-glycemic cupcakes do exist in the form of these lemon-scented treats. The almond meal and coconut flour give you a wonderful way to have your cake and eat it, too! Crystallized maple syrup presented as "sugar crystals" can be substituted for the pure maple syrup. You can find it in the baking section of your local market or at an artisanal food store.

CUPCAKES:

- ¼ cup plus 3 tablespoons extra-virgin coconut oil
- 5 large eggs
- 1 teaspoon pure vanilla extract
- ⅛ teaspoon sea salt
- 2 tablespoons pure maple syrup
- 1 tablespoon pure lemon extract
- ½ teaspoon baking powder
- 2 tablespoons almond meal
- ¼ cup plus 2 tablespoons coconut flour

DARK CHOCOLATE AVOCADO ICING (OPTIONAL):

- flesh of 2 avocados
- ½ cup unsweetened cocoa powder
- 1 tablespoon maple sugar
- ⅓ cup agave nectar
- ½ teaspoon pure vanilla extract
- 1 tablespoon unsweetened almond milk
- 1 tablespoon coconut butter

MAKE THE CUPCAKES:

1. Preheat the oven to 400°F. Line a 24-cup mini muffin pan with 20 baking cups and grease the cups with 1 tablespoon of the coconut oil.

2. In a medium bowl mix the eggs, vanilla, salt, maple syrup, lemon extract, and baking powder with an electric hand mixer on medium-high speed.

3. Add the almond meal, coconut flour, and remaining ¼ cup plus 2 tablespoons coconut oil and blend with the mixer until no lumps of flour remain.

4. Fill the baking cups three-quarters of the way to the top with batter. Give the pan a few gentle taps on the counter to remove any air trapped in the batter and slide the pan into the oven on the middle rack. Bake until a toothpick comes out clean when inserted into the center of the cupcakes, about 10 minutes. Cool in the pan for 5 minutes. Transfer to a wire rack to cool for another 10 minutes before topping with the icing, if using.

MAKE THE ICING:

Combine all of the icing ingredients in a food processor and blend until smooth.

Nutritional analysis per serving (1 cupcake without icing): calories 68, fat 5 g, saturated fat 4 g, cholesterol 37 mg, fiber 1 g, protein 2 g, carbohydrate 3 g, sodium 30 mg

Nutritional analysis per serving (1 cupcake with icing): calories 128, fat 9 g, saturated fat 5 g, cholesterol 37 mg, fiber 3 g, protein 3 g, carbohydrate 11 g, sodium 32 mg

CHOCOLATE ZUCCHINI BREAD

Serves: 12

Prep time: 15 minutes

Cook time: 40 minutes

Level: Moderate

Budget: $$

Almond meal can be substituted for gluten-containing flours. This is a low-glycemic, high-protein bread with a sweet-sour taste from the cherries and chocolate. Coconut sugar, crystallized coconut sap, is gluten-free and has a lower glycemic load than cane sugar. You can buy roasted pecans, but if you roast at home you can control the heat in order to prevent oxidization of healthy fats and rancidity; heat pecans in toaster oven at 275°F for 3–5 minutes or until fragrant and slightly brown.

- 2 cups almond meal
- 2 ounces 70% dark chocolate, roughly chopped
- ½ cup ground roasted pecans
- ¼ cup coconut sugar
- ¼ cup unsweetened cocoa powder
- ¼ cup unsweetened coconut flakes
- ¼ cup dried sour cherries, roughly chopped
- 1 teaspoon ground cinnamon
- ½ teaspoon baking soda
- ½ teaspoon sea salt
- 2 large eggs
- ¼ cup coconut butter, melted
- 1 cup zucchini, grated

1. Preheat the oven to 325°F. Grease a 9-inch loaf pan and line it with parchment paper. Set aside.
2. Add all of the dry ingredients to the bowl of an electric stand mixer. Turn to low speed to combine everything evenly.
3. In a separate large bowl mix the eggs, coconut butter, and zucchini.
4. Add the wet ingredients to the dry ingredients and turn the mixer to medium speed. Mix for 2–3 minutes, then lift the paddle attachment and scrape down the sides of the work bowl to ensure there are no trapped patches of dry ingredients. Engage the paddle and turn the mixer on low to fold everything together for 10–15 seconds.

5. Spread the batter into the baking pan. Bake until a toothpick comes out clean when inserted into the center of the bread, 35–40 minutes. Cool for 10 minutes in the pan, then transfer to a wire rack and let it fully cool. Cut into 12 slices. The bread can be stored in the freezer for up to 3 months.

Nutritional analysis per serving (1 slice): calories 234, fat 19 g, saturated fat 3 g, cholesterol 27 mg, fiber 3.5 g, protein 6 g, carbohydrate 13 g, sodium 177 mg

Acknowledgments

Cooking has always been one of my deepest pleasures and a way to connect with something real, tangible, and creative. Cooking is a revolutionary act. And revolutions take many people. This cookbook grew out of the revolution brewing in our country of people who are bringing cooking and real, whole, fresh, delicious food back to the center of their lives and communities.

I believe the community, our communities, small and large are the cure for what ails us. So I called upon my community of readers to offer their favorite recipes that follow the guidelines from *The Blood Sugar Solution*. I was overwhelmed with submissions and picked the best for this cookbook. Without all of you, this cookbook would not have happened. I thank all the cooking revolutionaries out there who made this book possible.

And of course, this book would never have happened if it were not for the energy, vision, dedication, and passion of my team. Thank you all. Anne McLaughlin stands by and behind me in everything and anything and stitched together the whole cookbook almost singlehandedly from my sometimes chaotic visions and writings. Thank you!!! And Shibani Subramanya and Daffnee Cohen helped pull our community together into this wonderful book, and they support everything I do. Lizzy Swick, my loyal and dedicated nutritionist, oversaw the recipes, making sure they faithfully matched my demands for healing, taste, and fun. Jonathan Heindemause tested and improved on every recipe and took the mouthwatering photographs in the book.

And last but not least, I offer my deepest gratitude to my editor, Tracy Behar, and the team at Little, Brown for supporting my radical notion that we can transform health and healthcare and making this book a reality. And of course, Richard Pine, my agent, whose magic touch and vision make everything I do easier and more effective. Thank you for being there for me.

The Contributors:

Alison L.: Blissful Butternut Bisque, Dark Chocolate Almond–Butter Bark, Grapefruit and Avocado Salad with Dijon Lime Vinaigrette, Green Goddess Broccoli and Arugula Soup, Pesce al Cartoccio (Fish Baked in Parchment Paper)

Alyssa G.: Garden Omelet

Arti Rajvanshi: Quinoa-Bean-Vegetable Cutlets with Bean Sprouts and Cilantro Chutney

Audrey M.: Seasoned Kale

Auralee B.: Learn to Love Brussels Sprouts

BJ R.: End-of-the-Garden Zucchini Meal

Bonnie C.: Eggwich

Brandy A.: Brandy's Healthy Turkey–Pinto Bean Chili

Bridget T.: Asian Prawn Paella

Caroline Fortin: Almond-Crusted Salmon with Lentil Salad

Cathy O.: Soba Noodle Salad with Bok Choy

Cathy Sandfort: Roasted Apple and Sweet Potato Medley

Charla R.: Asian Lettuce Boats, Curried Winter Squash Soup

Christine B.: Make-Ahead Super Warm and Filling Breakfast

Cindy L.: Blue Cheese Cowboy Burger

Connie Eilers: Slow Cooker Vegetarian Chili

Danielle M.: Spiced Turkey Salad

Deana T.: Herbed Tomato Spread

Deborah C.: Quinoa with Citrus Vinaigrette

Diane E.: Guaco Tacos

Donna J.: Beef and Bean Tacos

Donna K.: Frozen Fun Pops, Pink Pom Pom

Elaine C.: Strawberry Ice Cream

Elisa H.: Berry Blast Chia Porridge with Hemp Milk

Ellen G.: Kale and Brussels Sprout Salad

Esme Greer: Gingered Chicken with Cashews, Carrots, Raisins, and Scallions

Esther Ordenes: Chile Verde Chicken

Esther W.: Grilled Mixed Vegetables

Evelyn R.: Spaghetti Squash Pad Thai

Experience Life: Crispy Kale Chips with Sea Salt

Gavin C.: Healthiest Breakfast in the World

Helena G.: Chocolate Chia Seed Pudding, Deluxe Guacamole, Guilt-Free Chocolate Mousse

Helena L.: Chocolate Nut Cake, Popeye the Sailor Energy Boost

Helmut Beierbeck: Chinese Fried Quinoa

Holly M.: Beef and Cabbage Casserole

Ilona E.: Asian Quinoa Salad

Jamie P.: Five Taste Senses in One Perfect Bite

Jane Campbell: Dandelion Dip

Janine S.: Spicy Salmon Salad

Janis S.: Roasted Veggie and Chicken Chopped Salad

Jayme Goffin: Spicy Sage Turkey Sausage

Jean R.: Sautéed Spinach and Tomatoes over Roasted Spaghetti Squash

Jeanne R.: Black Bean Tofu Salad

Jeni C.: Addictive Creamy Garlic Dressing

Jennifer B.: Texas-Style Turkey Chili

Jennifer J.: Dark Chocolate Silk Pudding

Jessica Mishra: Healing Chicken Soup, Kale with Carrots and Arame

Judy R.: Almond-Crusted Chicken Breasts, Baked Salmon Cakes

Julie D.: Roasted Veggies to Make Your Liver Happy

Julie G.: Latin Black Bean Burgers

Karen Heringer: Chocolate Zucchini Bread

Karen S.: Karen's Southwest Black Bean Soup, Raw Chocolate Protein Shake, Spicy Black Bean Burgers

Kim T.: Chickpea and Kale Salad

Kimberly B.: Green Egg Skillet Bake, Roasted Chicken and Egg White Cup

Kristen M.: Kristen's Kale Waldorf

Kristy M.: Nutty Salmon Salad

Lara Zakaria: Wild Rice and Salmon with Collards

Laurie B.: Shirataki Noodles with Kale and Chickpeas

Leslie Keegan : Raspberry Banana Cream Pie Smoothie

Lidia L.: Green Chia Porridge

Linda Arndt: Chicken Salvatore

Linda M.: Chunky Avocado Tacos

Linda V.: Lemony Greek Pan-Roasted Chickpeas

Lisa B.: Double Peanut Butter Chocolate Cups

Lisa Beach: Coconut-Flour Flatbread Sandwich, Lisa's Lemon Vanilla Cupcakes

Lisa C.: Salmon Party Pâté

Lisa H.: Broccoli Scramble

Lisa M.: Lisa's Famous Guacamole

Lon W.: Summer Salad

Lorraine C.: Blueberry Muffins

Maggie S.: Weekday Veggie Scramble

Margaret F.: Bean Salad

Marilyn C.: Curried Cream of Cauliflower Soup

Marsha B.: Curried Spinach with Chickpeas and Coconut Milk

Mary T.: Sweet Potato Burgers

Maureen W.: Kickin' Kale Salad

Michael S.: Mighty "Meaty" Meatless Stew

Michele R.: Creamy Asparagus Soup

Michele R.: Roasted Red Pepper and Cannellini Bean Soup

Mona S.: Spiced Ground Turkey Wrap with Watercress and Avocado

Murthy S.: Bean Soup

Nathalie Fraise: Cashew Cheese

Noreen A.: Southwestern Chicken and Vegetable Soup

Pam B.: Pam's Delicious and Healthy Vegetable Stir-Fry

Pam S.: Strawberry Spinach Salad

Phyllis T.: Shrimp Salsa

Rebecca F.: Edamame Bean Salad, Ginger Edamame Salad

Rivkah B.: Vegan Lasagna

Ruth Rosenberg: Mom's Poached Fish in Velvety Tomato Sauce

Sally C.: Vegetable Chili with Smoked Spices

Sam S.: Roasted Cauliflower

Sandra R.: Mexican Lasagna

Sara S.: Hearty Greens with Ginger and Sugar Snap Peas over Soba

Sheila C.: Tuscan Zucchini Soup

Sheila Ternovacz: Mexican Shrimp "Ceviche"

Shelly J.: Spicy Triple Green Sauté

Sheri Dixon: Sadie's White Bean and Shrimp Soup

Sheri M.: Hearty Lentil Soup

Sona N.: Asian Coleslaw

Sorina B.: Red Cabbage Salad

Susan Sahlgren: Hearty Kale Vegetable Stew

Sylvia Alakusheva: Quinoa and Avocado Salad

Tiffany L.: Matcha Green Energizer

Todd S.: Cauliflower Mashed Pseudo-Potatoes

Tracy B.: Guilt-Free Cauliflower Pizza Bites

Tracy K.: Cilantro, Edamame, and Pine Nut Salad

Tracy Keibler: Spicy Chicken Stir-Fry

Tracy S.: Slow-Baked Salmon

Valerie M.: Special Beans and Greens

Resources

Mark Hyman's Websites
www.drhyman.com
www.bloodsugarsolution.com
www.takebackourhealth.org
www.ultramind.com

The UltraWellness Center
55 Pittsfield Road, Suite 9
Lenox Commons
Lenox, MA 01240
(413) 637-9991
www.ultrawellnesscenter.com
Our team of experienced functional medicine physicians, nutritionists, nurses, and health coaches guide you through diet and lifestyle modifications, as well as specialized testing, nutritional supplementation, and medications to address the root causes of chronic disease.

The Blood Sugar Solution (the book)
www.bloodsugarsolution.com
In *The Blood Sugar Solution,* I reveal that the secret solution to losing

weight and preventing not just diabetes but also heart disease, stroke, dementia, and cancer is balanced insulin levels. I describe the seven keys to achieving wellness — nutrition, hormones, inflammation, digestion, detoxification, energy metabolism, and a calm mind — and explain my revolutionary six-week healthy-living program. With advice on diet, green living, supplements and medication, exercise, and personalizing the plan for optimal results, the book also teaches readers how to maintain lifelong health. Groundbreaking and timely, the Blood Sugar Solution is the fastest way to lose weight, prevent disease, and feel better than ever.

The Blood Sugar Solution PBS Special

www.bloodsugarsolution.com/pbs

In this 60-minute program, I explain what "diabesity" is, outline the underlying causes that drive the problem, and provide a personalized, 4-step plan to help you overcome diabesity. I also explain how we can all take back our health as individuals, as a community, and as a society.

The program will radically change the way you think about your body, your lifestyle, and the power you have to change your health. I identify the seven keys to achieving wellness and outline the steps needed to personalize your approach to healing. My six-week action plan will help you identify and address the unique causes of your own health and weight issues, and I offer exercise advice, stress-reducing strategies, a menu plan with delicious recipes, and much more.

The UltraMind Solution (the book)

www.bloodsugarsolution.com/ultramind-solution

Whether you suffer from a mood disorder, neurological problems, difficulty with attention, low energy, or brain fog, this six-week program will help to heal your brain by fixing your body first.

The UltraMind Solution PBS Special

www.bloodsugarsolution.com/ultramind-dvd

Learn about the seven key systems that are at the root of all broken brains, and what you can do to live a vibrantly healthy life.

Six Weeks to an UltraMind (the audio/DVD program)

www.bloodsugarsolution.com/six-weeks-to-ultramind

This dynamic self-coaching program provides a combination of audio, video, and printed materials that make incorporating the UltraMind program into your life as simple as possible.

UltraCalm (the audio program)

www.bloodsugarsolution.com/ultracalm

Are you stressed out? Do you suffer from anxiety, obsessive-compulsive disorders, or panic attacks? In this audio program, I walk you through steps you can take to help you resolve stress and anxiety. It includes guided visualizations, breathing exercises, tips on nutrition, detoxification, and more.

UltraMetabolism (the book)

www.bloodsugarsolution.com/ultrametabolism

This book promises to reprogram your body to automatically lose weight by turning on the messages of weight loss and health and turning off the messages of weight gain and disease.

The UltraMetabolism PBS Special

www.bloodsugarsolution.com/ultrametabolism-dvd

This two-hour special brings the secrets and steps of the UltraMetabolism program home.

The UltraMetabolism Cookbook

www.bloodsugarsolution.com/ultrametabolism-cookbook

This book provides 200 recipes to put the UltraMetabolism program into overdrive. They are also great for the Blood Sugar Solution.

The UltraSimple Diet (the book)

www.bloodsugarsolution.com/ultrasimple-diet

This simple seven-day program provides the tools you need to treat the two primary underlying factors of weight gain—toxins and inflammation—and not only lose weight but also alleviate many of your chronic health symptoms.

The UltraSimple Challenge

www.bloodsugarsolution.com/ultrasimple-challenge

- DVD Coaching Program. Two DVDs include information on why and how the program works, the science behind it, daily motivational and instructional videos, and a special section on how to keep the weight off and the health on for good.
- 7-Day Action Plan Guide. This includes meal plans, shopping lists, recommended supplements, exercises and relaxation techniques, daily checklists, food logs, a journal, and progress trackers.
- Online Support Community. Connect with other people on the program and share your experiences. Community support is a critical factor in making long-term changes.

The UltraThyroid Solution (the ebook)

www.bloodsugarsolution.com/ultrathyroid

Learn the seven steps that will help you comprehensively address your low-functioning thyroid and heal from this potentially devastating disorder.

UltraPrevention (the book)

www.bloodsugarsolution.com/ultraprevention

This includes an innovative program that shatters the myths of today's "fix the broken parts" medicine.

Five Forces of Wellness (the audio program)

www.bloodsugarsolution.com/5forces

Learn about the five imbalances that lead to disease and how you can turn them into the five forces of wellness instead.

The Detox Box
www.bloodsugarsolution.com/detoxbox
This program is designed to remove toxins and allergens, boost immunity, and restore energy. The box includes CDs, flash cards, and a quick-start guide to give you everything you need to complete a safe, effective, and medically informed detoxification program at home.

Nutrigenomics
www.bloodsugarsolution.com/nutrigenomics
Find out which foods you can use to leverage your body's natural ability to heal itself.

FOOD RESOURCES

Here you'll find a vast array of organic foods; home care, health care, kitchenware, and pet care products; as well as other valuable resources.

Organic Essentials

The Organic Pages
www.bloodsugarsolution.com/theorganicpages
The Organic Trade Association (OTA) provides users with a quick and easy way to find certified organic products, producers, ingredients, supplies, and services offered by OTA members, as well as items of interest to the entire organic community.

Organic Planet
www.bloodsugarsolution.com/organic-planet
Organic Planet is a leading supplier of natural and organic food ingredients.

Organic Provisions
www.bloodsugarsolution.com/orgfood

Organic Provisions is a convenient new way of choosing a wide array of quality natural foods and products right from your home.

Sun Organic Farm
www.bloodsugarsolution.com/sunorganicfarm
Sun Organic Farm provides a direct source for online ordering of a wide variety of organic foods.

Produce

Earthbound Farm
www.ebfarm.com
Offers fresh, packaged organic produce.

Maine Coast Sea Vegetables
www.bloodsugarsolution.com/seaveg
A variety of sea vegetables, including some organically certified types.

Organic Frozen and Canned Foods

Cascadian Farm
www.bloodsugarsolution.com/cfarm
A great source of organic frozen fruit and vegetables for those in a hurry.

Imagine Foods
www.bloodsugarsolution.com/imaginefoods
A high-quality purveyor of delicious organic soups.

Pacific Foods
www.bloodsugarsolution.com/pacificfoods
Pacific Foods carries high-quality soups, broths, nut milk, hemp milk, and more.

Stahlbush Island Farms

www.bloodsugarsolution.com/stahlbush

An excellent source of sustainably grown frozen berries.

Meat, Poultry, Eggs, and Dairy

Applegate Farms

www.bloodsugarsolution.com/applegatefarms

Packaged poultry, meat, and deli products.

Eatwild

www.bloodsugarsolution.com/eatwild

Grass-fed meat and dairy products.

Organic Valley

www.bloodsugarsolution.com/organicvalley

Organic meats, dairy, eggs, and produce from more than 600 member-owned organic farms.

Peaceful Pastures

www.bloodsugarsolution.com/peacefulpastures

Grass-fed and grass-finished meat, poultry, and dairy products.

Pete and Gerry's Organic Eggs

www.bloodsugarsolution.com/peteandgerrys

Organic omega-3 eggs.

Stonyfield

www.bloodsugarsolution.com/stonyfield

Certified organic dairy products and soy yogurt.

Fish

Clean Fish
www.cleanfish.com
A wonderful resource for sustainably caught or farmed fish.

Crown Prince Natural
www.bloodsugarsolution.com/crownprince
Wild-caught, sustainably harvested, specialty canned seafood.

EcoFish
www.bloodsugarsolution.com/ecofish
Environmentally responsible seafood products and information.

SeaBear
www.bloodsugarsolution.com/seabear
Wild salmon jerky for a convenient snack.

Vital Choice
www.bloodsugarsolution.com/vitalchoice
A selection of fresh, frozen, and canned wild salmon, sardines, black cod, and small halibut.

Nuts, Seeds, and Oils

Artisana Foods
www.artisanafoods.com
My favorite source of nut butter and coconut butter.

Barlean's Organic Oils
www.bloodsugarsolution.com/barleans
Organic oils and ground flaxseeds.

Maranatha

www.bloodsugarsolution.com/worldpantry

Organic nut and seed butters.

Omega Nutrition

www.bloodsugarsolution.com/omeganutrition

A variety of organic oils, flax, and hemp seed products.

Once Again

www.bloodsugarsolution.com/onceagainnutbutter

Organic nut and seed butters.

Spectrum Naturals

www.bloodsugarsolution.com/spectrumorganic

An extensive line of high-quality oils, vinegars, flaxseed products, and culinary resources.

Beans and Legumes

Eden Foods

www.bloodsugarsolution.com/edenfoods

A complete line of organic dried and canned beans.

Westbrae Natural

www.bloodsugarsolution.com/westbrae

A full variety of organic beans and vegetarian products (soups, condiments, pastas, etc.)

Grains

Arrowhead Mills

www.bloodsugarsolution.com/arrowheadmills

Organic grains, including many gluten-free choices.

Hodgson Mill
www.bloodsugarsolution.com/hodgsonmill
A complete line of whole grains, including many gluten-free grains.

Lundberg Family Farms
www.bloodsugarsolution.com/lundberg
Organic grains and gluten-free items, such as wild rice.

Shiloh Farms
www.bloodsugarsolution.com/shilohfarms
Organic whole grains, sprouted grains, and gluten-free items.

Spices, Seasonings, Sauces, Soups, and Such

Edward & Sons
www.bloodsugarsolution.com/edwardandsons
An extensive line of vegetarian organic food products including miso, sauces, brown rice crackers, etc.

Flavorganics
www.bloodsugarsolution.com/flavorganics
A full product line of certified organic pure flavor extracts.

Frontier Natural Products Co-Op
www.bloodsugarsolution.com/frontiernaturalbrands
An extensive line of organic spices, seasonings, baking flavors and extracts, dried foods, teas, and culinary gadgets.

Rapunzel
www.bloodsugarsolution.com/rapunzel
A great selection of seasonings such as Herbamare, made with sea salt and organic herbs.

Seeds of Change
www.bloodsugarsolution.com/seedsofchange
Organic tomato sauce, salsa, and more.

Spice Hunter
www.bloodsugarsolution.com/spicehunter
A complete line of organic spices.

Nondairy, Gluten-Free Beverages

Soy Dream
www.bloodsugarsolution.com/tastethedream
Soy and rice milk and ice creams.

Westbrae WestSoy
www.bloodsugarsolution.com/westsoy
Unsweetened soy milk.

WhiteWave
www.bloodsugarsolution.com/silksoymilk
Silk soy milk beverage.

WholeSoy & Co.
www.bloodsugarsolution.com/wholesoyco
Unsweetened soy yogurt.

Organic Herbal Teas

Choice Organic Teas
www.bloodsugarsolution.com/choiceorganicteas
Organic fair-trade teas.

Mighty Leaf Tea
www.bloodsugarsolution.com/mightyleaf
Artisan-crafted loose teas in biodegradable pouches.

Numi Tea
www.bloodsugarsolution.com/numitea
Numi inspires well-being of mind, body, and spirit through the simple art of tea.

Yogi Tea
www.bloodsugarsolution.com/yogitea
Medicinal herbal teas.

Water

The best water filters are reverse osmosis filters. While they can be more expensive, the investment is worth it as they remove more toxins from your water supply. If your budget won't allow reverse osmosis filters, Brita is a good alternative.

Reverse-Osmosis Filters
www.bloodsugarsolution.com/h2odistributors

Brita
www.bloodsugarsolution.com/brita

General Index

Note: Italic page numbers refer to tables.

Recipe Index

About the Author

Mark Hyman, MD, has dedicated his career to identifying and addressing the root causes of chronic illness through a groundbreaking whole-systems medicine approach known as Functional Medicine. He is a family physician, a five-time #1 *New York Times* bestselling author, and an internationally recognized leader in his field. Through his private practice, education efforts, writing, research, advocacy, and public-policy work, he strives to improve access to and expand the practice of Functional Medicine, empowering others to treat the underlying causes of illness, tackling the roots of our chronic-disease epidemic.

Dr. Hyman is Chairman of the Institute for Functional Medicine, and was awarded its 2009 Linus Pauling Award for Leadership in Functional Medicine. He is also on the Advisory Board of *The Dr. Oz Show* and on the Board of Advisors of Mehmet Oz's HealthCorps, which tackles the obesity epidemic by educating the student body in American high schools about nutrition, fitness, and mental resilience. Dr. Hyman is on the board of the Center for Mind Body Medicine and the board of the Environmental Working Group.

He has testified before the Senate Working Group on Health Care Reform on Functional Medicine and, in June 2009, he participated in the White House Forum on Prevention and Wellness. Dr. Hyman was nominated by Senator Tom Harkin for the President's Advisory Group on Prevention, Health Promotion, and Integrative and Public Health, a 25-person group to advise the Administration and the new National Council on Prevention, Health Promotion, and Public Health. With Drs. Dean Ornish and Michael Roizen, Dr. Hyman crafted and helped to introduce the *Take Back Your Health Act of 2009* into the United States Senate, to provide for reimbursement of lifestyle treatment of chronic disease.

Through his work with corporations, church groups, and government entities, such as CIGNA, the Veterans Administration, Google, Saddleback Church, and the World Economic Forum, he is helping to improve health outcomes and reduce costs around the world. He initiated and is a key participant in the ongoing development of a faith-based initiative that enrolled over 15,000 people at Saddleback Church in a healthy lifestyle program and research study. In one year they lost 250,000 pounds based on the principles of the Blood Sugar Solution. Please join him in helping us all take back our health at www.drhyman.com, and follow him on Twitter @markhymanmd and on Facebook at facebook.com/drmarkhyman.

3 1901 05433 0693